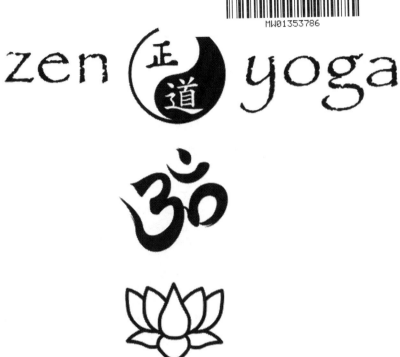

Theory, Postures & Remedies

By Colleen Inman

Zenspirations
Phoenix, Arizona

Disclaimer

This book is intended for information purposes only. The author and publisher do not promise or imply any results to those using this information, nor are they responsible for any negative results brought about by the usage of the information contained herein.

The author and publisher of this book and the accompanying materials have used their best efforts in preparing this book. The author and publisher make no representation of warranties with respect to the accuracy, applicability, fitness, or completeness of the contents of this book. Furthermore, the author and publisher do not guarantee that the holder of this information will improve his or her health from the information contained herein.

Each individual's health will be determined by his or her desire, dedication, background, effort, motivation to practice and follow the program, and his or her current health conditions. There is no guarantee you will duplicate the results stated here. You recognize that health programs are dependent on many factors to be successful.

Copyright © 2015 by Colleen Inman.

All rights reserved. No part of this book may be reproduced or used in any form or by any means, electronic or mechanical, including photocopying, recording, or by any information storage and retrieval system, without prior written permission from the author and Zenspirations LLC.

ISBN-13: 978-1-5194-7648-7
ISBN-10: 1-5194-7648-5

Zenspirations LLC
www.scwzenwellness.com
colleen@zenwellness.com

Dedication

For my sons Luca and Michael.

Much gratitude to those who have contributed to this work. To Master Jason Campbell and Master Michael J. Leone, who both helped with the content, because of their ongoing instruction, support, and input, these teachings have an opportunity to live on.

Thank you to everyone who has supported and enhanced my journey. My sister Ashley, my son Luca, my father, John, teachers Debbie Forrest, Kat Myers, Beth Hayes-Leone, Grand Master Stuart Alve Olson, Grand Master Sung Baek, Grand Master Puquan Xiao, Master Sara Anderson, and John Friend to name a few.

Grateful for the information age we live in, where "Grand Master Google" has been there 24/7 giving endless information and fact checking abilities. To Patrick Gross for taking on the task of editing and typesetting the book.

Thank you to all the human beings who have studied the lineages and took the time to pay it forward, write it down, and make teachings available to the masses.

Contents

Introduction 1

Part 1: Staying Well 3

Part 2: The Alchemy of Yin-Yang 7

Part 3: Three Levels of Consciousness 23

Part 4: The Four Pillars 29

Part 5: Balancing the Elements 33

Part 6: Prana/Qi—The Sixth Element 59

Part 7: The Seven Chakras 63

Part 8: Eight Trigrams, Eight Vessels, Eight Limbs of Yoga 77

Part 9: Nine Gates & Three Hearts 109

Part 10: Asanas (Postures) 119

Part 11: Pranayama (Qi Gong Breath Work) 221

Part 12: Nadis/Meridians, The Horary Cycle/
Astrological Twelve 235

Introduction
What Is Zen Yoga?

"Zen" is an approach or method in which something is done. Zen implies simply constantly residing in the present moment.

"Yoga" is derived from the Sanskrit root *yuj,* meaning to "bind, join, attach and yoke," "union," to direct and concentrate one's attention on us, and "apply." Yoga is the act of unifying one's mind, physical body and energy body in a balanced manner.

"Zen Yoga" offers a seeker of a balanced self a proven method in which to obtain such a union. Zen blossomed around 2,600 years ago as a method to solve the problem of human suffering through calming of the mind. The union of Yoga harmonizes the physical body and energy body, creating a sense of balance that leaves one in good health.

To be without suffering implies to be in good order; this is accomplished only after the mind is at ease, the physical body is without pain, and the energy body glows without blockages.

Zen Yoga incorporates *asanas* (postures) to first restore, then strengthen, and finally expand the seeker's physical anatomy. "Flexible body, flexible mind."

Zen Yoga then teaches the energetic anatomy of oneself so the seeker may actively participate in balancing optimal circulation of energy around the physical body's space.

Zen Yoga seekers use the lessons of "Zen" to quiet the mind.

These three harmonies allow the clarity of the seeker's higher self to show up and lead one's way (destiny).

In studying the art of Zen Yoga, you will be introduced to ideas found in multiple cultures with the understanding that *"What is true is true for all, or not at all."* For humanity to resolve human suffering, the adherent to one culture or belief must merge and pan out to a larger view of humanity as a whole. As one begins to see that although we might be titled "American," "Chinese," or "African," we all fit in to the general title of "Earthling." Each culture has "believed truths," however, the "certain truths" are the ones that are true for everyone no matter a country's borders. Gravity, for example, is equally true for everyone. It doesn't change at any border, or is affected by your social status, or even by the God to whom you pray. Gravity is simply gravity.

Zen Yoga encourages a seeker to step back from one's myopic view and see the bigger picture. Do this by examining the root teachings that are common in many wisdom traditions. In examining different wisdom traditions, commonalities can be seen in their usage of numbers. For instance, 0 = nothingness, 1 = consciousness within; 2 = yin/yang or polarity; 3 = three levels of being; 5 = elements; 7 = chakras, dimensions, and levels of heaven; 8 = energetic behaviors; 12 = meridians and astrology. Zen Yoga explores these common traits as pointers for optimal living and co-existence.

There is no need to renounce your current beliefs or ideologies. Hopefully, you will shed a light of consciousness to see the truths in your current traditions so as to strengthen your beliefs by seeing how they fit in the larger picture.

Zen Yoga is calling your higher self to your mat. Are you listening?

Part 1
Staying Well

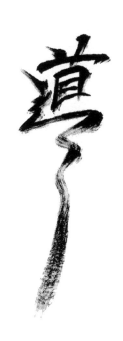

Balanced Mind, Physical Body and Energetic Body

is the method of staying well. We know today that stress is one of the most common factors in sickness and dis-ease. When cells are stressed the structure of the cell walls change and become inconsistent sizes and shapes, often from inflammation. Imagine the walls, roof and foundation of your house changing shape and size—what would happen? The reasons for which the house was built (to provide shelter from the environment and pests) no longer functions properly. Apply this idea to the cells in your body. They are designed to keep a specific shape and size so as to work properly keeping in "good stuff" and keeping out "bad invaders" or external pathogens.

Staying well does not imply there will be an absence of stress factors in your reality, instead it points to your ability to manage and not get caught up in the story of your stresses, constantly watching your mind.

Physical actions of staying well include moving the body in specific ways to flush out old decaying matter and excess heat or inflammation held within the body. Proper movement of the physical body includes consideration of age, past activities, and honoring current limitations. When exercising or moving the physical body, temperature is the first consideration. Within the body is a lymphatic system responsible for removing problematic material. When working out at high pace and overheating the body, the lymph system responds by temporarily shutting down (it thinks you are running from a tiger and need all energy and blood for fight or flight). The key is to slowly warm the body and use slow steady fluid movements to assist the lymphatic system's process. Thus the wellness practices of yoga, qigong, and tai chi reduce the effects of age by removing waste and cooling inflammation. Staying well is staying young.

Taoist Immortality

Grandmaster Sung Baek, one of my teachers on Taoist Immortality—which is about not necessarily living forever, yet living fully while in this body—puts it like this. He uses the analogy of the body being like a sword blade, and says, "If you have a sword that is a few hundred years old but has never been polished, it will be old and rusty. But what if you cleaned and sharpened it every day? The blade would then be sharp and shine brightly. It is the same with your body and your health. Polish your 'blade' daily and you can stay strong as you age."

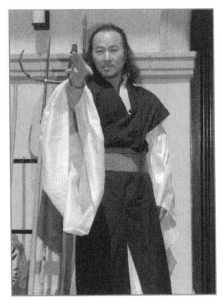

Grandmaster Sung Baek

Part 2

The Alchemy of Yin-Yang

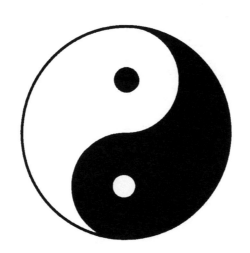

Wuji

Infinite consciousness with the compressing desire to experience itself contracts, creating a vacuum until it is strong enough to pull matter through its central void and explode matter into the womb space of itself. The empty comment bubble represents a Wuji field in which an infinite potential things may appear—words, exclamations, symbols, pictures … you name it. The thought projected into the field is the yang portion of the expression. Thus, the white yang bubble is inside a yin dark-square container. Without the white bubble inside, nothing would exist—this is wuji.

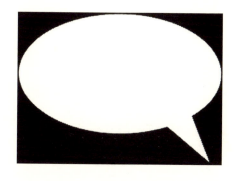

Once the polarity of the white bubble is established, yin and yang are born. Then again, once the full black square is filled with the yang spark of consciousness, it soon flips to become a yin container in which future images or words will appear.

The compression inside the womb space presses the matter together with force until the material has no choice but to combine and create a new form of matter. This process is expressed in the formation of the periodic table of elements. Starting with hydrogen and finishing its ability to compress at iron, thus creating the opposition of experiencing formless consciousness expressed in creation of formed consciousness, or the polarity of non-existence and existence.

> *The Tao that can be described is not the eternal Tao. The name that can be spoken is not the eternal Name. The nameless is the boundary of Heaven and Earth. The named is the mother of creation. Freed from desire, you can see the hidden mystery.*

> *By having desire, you can only see what is visibly real. Yet mystery and reality emerge from the same source. This source is called emptiness (no-thing). No-thing born from no-thing. The beginning of all understanding.*
>
> —Lao Tzu, 500 BCE

What Is Prana?

The animating force of life's expressions would be *Prana* (aka *Qi*). Prana is movement, and movement is prana. The cause and effect is prana. Prana is the animating life force within any living thing. Translated as "natural energy," "qi," "life force energy," "breath of life," "vital energy," "mana" or "the force." The Chinese character is a symbol of a cooking pot of rice with steam rising. The 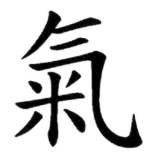 steam is "qi." The art of manipulating prana is the foundational practice of all the wisdom paradigms of yoga, qigong, tai chi, kung fu, acupuncture, chakra work, and so on. The "Prana" within living things expresses the vitality or light in the individual life form showing in its movement abilities (range of motion and stability), timing of reactions, and sense awareness. Prana is represented in one's breath on a cold day, smoke, steam, and other vapors, such as the visible upward moving heat off hot summer asphalt, cars, and desert landscapes. The energetic phenomenon that is an entity of a business, home, or ghost.

Within the human body, prana is said to have many major functions: prana protects the body from disease, supports and sustains all movements, supports the body's transformation, retains fundamental substance and maintains normal body heat.

Part 2: The Alchemy of Yin-Yang

Theories of Traditional Indian and Chinese Medicine assert that the body has natural patterns of prana that circulate in channels called meridians and vessels. In Sanskrit these channels are called *nadis*. Symptoms of various illnesses are often believed to be the product of disrupted, blocked or unbalanced qi movement (interrupted flow) through the body's meridians, vessels and nadis, as well as deficiencies or imbalances of qi (homeostatic imbalance) in the various yin/yang (zang-fu) organs. Zen Yoga often seeks to relieve these imbalances by adjusting the circulation of qi in the body using a variety of Zen Yoga therapeutic techniques.

The Zen Yoga system has its roots in Taoist alchemy and Western science. Taoists have been responsible for advancing the development of gunpowder, herbology and acupuncture to name a few of their accomplishments. The Taoists see the creation of the universe beginning with wuji or ultimate stillness. Creation brings forth yin qi, yang qi and yuan qi, also known as positive, negative and neutral chi. These are transformed into each other in an eternal cycle of movement. This cycle of eternal movement is referred to as Tai Chi, which generates the five elements. The Five Elements form the universe, Milky Way, earth, man and the ten thousand things of life.

You can see these findings mirrored in Western science where positive, negative and neutral energy are bound together within each atom and are the building blocks of all things. Simply put, qi is this bio-magnetic energy that is within all living things. Where there is qi, there is life. When you are born you have an abundance of qi. The goal of Qigong (Chi Kung) is maintaining the abundance of qi and ensuring its proper circulation throughout the body.

Yin Yang

Theorem of opposites. Yin and yang are two of many words used to point at the perceived conception of duality. All cultures and wisdom teachings throughout time have done the best they can to explain the polarity of existence from non-existence. Some cultures simply use non-animated verbiage, while others personify deities through mythology to point at the inherent polar opposites.

Examples of non-animated verbiage opposites include yin and yang, up and down, in and out, right and left, and so on. Examples of animating yin/yang are done in ways to which we can humanly relate—Shiva/Shakti, Jesus/Mary Magdalene, Lilith/Chiron, Adam/Eve, Samson/Delilah, Persephone/Hades, Rama/Sita, Father Heaven/Mother Earth—all of which have many faces or sides to their persona.

Now having living and inanimate examples of the yin/yang duality, the relationships can be observed. Since yin/yang is a whole spinning idea of an entity starting, balancing, and duplicating, observing the pattern in which it transforms is important.

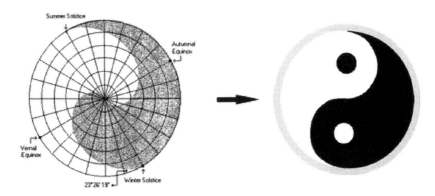

Above we see the two opposites. Black and white establish the polarity spoken of in the spark that illuminated in wuji. Yin and yang expresses in every asana (posture) in directing contracting and expanding principles. Imagine a tree using effort to root downward and grace in blossoming upward. Drilling into the earth and flowering upward to the heavens allows one to connect to both energies of heaven and earth and become a clean conduit for the two to meet and blend. This is the alchemy of Zen Yoga.

Within yin and yang are yin of yin, yin of yang, yang of yin, and yang of yang—symbolizing the in-between states of yin and yang. There is full yin—total darkness and full form; and there is full yang—total light and emptiness. However, there must be an account for middle ground, the gray area where the two meet and become the other. For example:

High noon (yang) and **midnight** (yin).
The gray area in between—sunrise (yang of yin)
and sunset (yin of yang).

Form (yin) and **emptiness** (yang).
Within form there is space (yang),
within emptiness is the womb (yin) for potential.

Cold (yin) and **hot** (yang).
Extreme cold can burn (yang),
extreme heat gives one the chills (yin)

Yin and yang always require an opposite for comparison. A tiger alone is neither yin nor yang. Compared to a rabbit, however, the tiger is yang. Compared to a T-Rex, it would be yin, so the qualification of something as yin or yang should be seen as a moving target. This brings up the first law of order in yin and yang theory.

The law of opposition. In order to exist (stand out), there must be a stated opposite. As babies our differences are minimal. It is not until later in childhood towards adolescence that one begins to stand on one side of the polarity. This polarity creates a charge—the male/female charge. In youth, one revels in its polarity and teases the opposite. When the teen years arrive, the understanding of the polarities existence is necessary. Thus the second law.

Law of inter-dependance. A new knowing develops that in order to exist, the polarity must be seen and present. Now through trial and error, couples form seeking the correct balanced fit. When a match becomes apparent, the third law follows.

Law of inter-consumption now comes into play. The couple begins to consume each other's time, energy, and space. Closing out the polarity of differences and making one unit who moves together sharing more and more of their time, energy, and space.

The **Law of Inter-transformation** arrives once the couple has completed the transformation of two separate existences (or lives) into one. Always showing up together as a united front. Once the gap has closed, the mated pair spawns another life form (either figuratively as in an incarnation of the couple's life together, or literally as in offspring) completing the yin-yang cycle with the **Law of Infinite Divisibility**.

Blending the theorem of yin and yang into one's practice often begins in the physical body, and ends in the consciousness or mind's understanding. Understanding that the relationship of yin and yang represents health is imperative in any seeker's path to deeper knowing. How else would one be able to see the in-dwelling spirit within as separate from the physical body?

Yin and Yang in Relation to Teaching

1. Class theme
2. Asana (posture)
3. Sequence

Class Theme

Each student seeks balance on some level when entering the practice room. The seat of the teacher is to hold the teacher space and guide the practitioner on his or her path by setting a theme or intention to focus on during the asanas. Theming offers contemplation of yin and yang from many angles or definitions.

Keeping to an intention of yin and yang promotes clarity to find balance. Examples of focusing on rooting and blossoming express the entire process, striking harmony and balance when the entire view becomes available, no matter if you are keeping this in mind simply for yourself or taking others through a practice. The class theme is set during the centering portion of a class, and brought back into the front of the mind multiple times throughout the practice.

Yin/Yang theme examples:

Expanding/Contracting	Effort/Ease
Action/Surrender	Power/Grace
Strength/Softness	Inflow/Outflow
Tapas/Ishwara-Pranidhana	

Asana

Each class should offer the student the opportunity to embody the yin/yang theme on a physical level. Describing how one might use the theme while working through an asana is the work of the teacher (either an actual teacher or the one within yourself). Example: Contemplate using contraction by drawing into the core then expanding the mind outward through the tips of your extremities.

Sequence

1. Centering (yin) to begin a class brings the practitioner inward (yin) from the outside world (yang).
2. Awakening with stretching and fluid movements.
3. Vitality comes from twisting to release blocked prana.
4. Equanimity to bring mental calmness and composure.
5. Grounding by developing root and lower body stability.

6. Igniting with dynamic back bends to release the fire contained within the heart.
7. Stability in building core.
8. Rejuvenation through inverting the physical body to optimize the flow of prana.
9. Releasing the spine with forward folds.
10. Surrender in savasana, letting go of life.

Zen Yoga: The Art of Teaching

Teaching is an art of communication.

If one teacher possesses 100 volts of knowledge but can effectively convey only 20 volts to his students, that teacher will be less effective than a teacher who combines 50 volts of knowledge with the ability to convey it all.

But, do not be overawed by win-loss records or lists of advanced degrees. What's important is not what teachers know, but what their students know; not what teachers can do but what their students can do.

Good teachers speak the language of the intellect—word—and communicate clearly so that students understand. They use hindsight to learn by their mistakes and improve.

Excellent teachers speak the language of the body—by showing muscles, bones and nerves how an activity should feel if done properly. They use foresight to anticipate the consequences of their actions.

Great teachers speak the language of the emotions—by inspiring, motivating, and encouraging a love of Yoga. They use insight to access the wisdom of the ages.

Master teachers do all three, using Yoga as a means to teach life.

—Dan Millman

On Teachers and Teaching

It is relatively easy to be a teacher of an academic subject, but to be a teacher in art is very difficult, and to be a yoga teacher is the hardest of all, because yoga teachers have to be their own critics and correct their own practice. The art of yoga is entirely subjective and practical. Yoga teachers have to know the entire functioning of the body; they have to know the behavior of the people who come to them and how to react and be ready to help, to protect and safeguard their pupils.

The requisites of a teacher are many, but I would like to give a few words for you all to catch, understand and work on. Later you can discover many more. The teacher should be clear, clever, confident, challenging, caring, cautious, constructive, courageous, comprehending, creative, completely devoted and dedicated to knowing the subject, considerate, conscientious, critical, committed, cheerful, chaste and calm. Teachers must be strong and positive in their approach. They must be affirmative to create confidence in the pupils, and navigate within themselves so that they can reflect critically on their own practice and attitudes. Teachers must always be learning. They will learn from the pupils and must have the humility to tell them that they are still learning their art.

—B.K.S. Iyengar

Mixing Kan & Li

Applying the alchemy of yin and yang through the art of yoga is the first action for the practitioner. Let's get to know the primary circuit of Zen Yoga ...

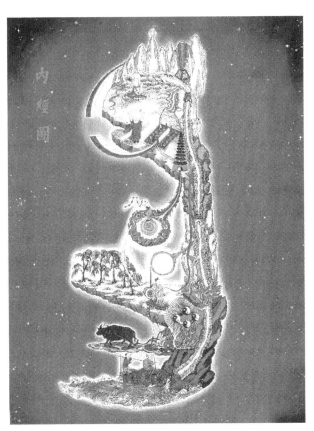

Small Circuit

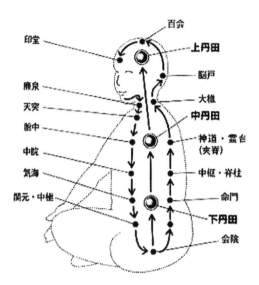

Now that you have been introduced to the concept of prana, the next step is to visualize the Hara or Brass Basin where you are creating what Taoists call the energy field elixir or lower dan tien. Then become aware of the Small Circuit. The Small Circuit has two major purposes: The first purpose is to build up prana at the lower dan tien, and the second is to store and circulate prana in the two major reservoirs, the Conception and Governing Vessels.

Then you must lead the prana through the vessels and open up the points that are blocked by mental, physical or emotional stress—the points running down the Conception Vessel (Ren Mai) or front of the body, and the points running up the Governing Vessel (Du Mai) or back of the body along the spine. Take time to visualize the points and commit them to memory. This will help when you start leading the prana through the Small Circuit with your lower abdominal breathing.

Small Circuit in Asana

Using small circuit visualization within asana practice physically opens the Governing and Conception channels to allow prana flow. Here we introduce the concepts of Kan and Li (Water and Fire). The mixing of Kan and Li is the single most profound piece of alchemy in the practice. The essential concept to all of life. One is to guide fire down the Conception Vessel, and send water up the Governing Vessel.

Tai Ji Pole/Sushumna Nadi

A vertical central primary energy vessel channeling qi from the root to crown chakra, housing each of the seven chakras and is surrounded by the three dan tiens. Considered the source of all prenatal life-force qi. A conduit running through humans connecting heaven and earth, called the Sushumna Nadi, Thrusting Vessel, and/or Tai Ji Pole. Mixing Ida and Pingala. The Tai Ji Pole is the third piece that prana will travel up after the small circuit.

Around the Sushumna Nadi circulates the Governing (along the back of the body) and Conception (along the front body) vessels. These vessels are used to descend heat downward (to warm the belly) and cool upward (to cool the head—no one likes a hot head).

The last two images of the *I Ching (Book of Changes)* speak to this concept with the images After Completion and Before Completion. When water is below fire there is no struggle, the water descends and the fire ascends and life is no more. However, when water is above fire then there is competition for the space. Water naturally falls and fire naturally rises, therefor they come to meet and create steam.

Two of the most commonly seen postures in yoga are Downward and Upward Facing Dog. These postures open the Governing (Downward Dog) and Conception (Upward Dog) vessels. In Zen Yoga, the exhale occurs with Upward Facing Dog to release fire-type energy stored in the the head and upper heart downward into the lower belly or low hara. The reverse posture, Downward Facing Dog offers lengthening of the spine to open the Governing Channel and allow the cool water naturally settled at the low back to move to the neck and head region to calm and cool the mind.

In studying the mixing of Kan & Li, balance is the goal. We start with balancing the fire and water energies in our body so we might begin to comprehend what these subtle concepts are, and then apply this knowledge to all areas of life.

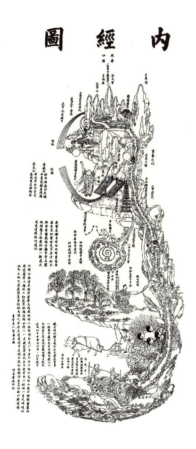

The image on the left is a classic Taoist diagram of the "Water Wheel." This diagram is one of many that could be found in ancient Taoist monasteries and temples. It depicts the inner energetic landscape and the mechanics of mixing Kan and Li.

Part 3

"OM"
The Three Levels of Consciousness

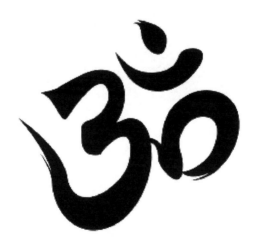

What Are the Three Levels of Consciousness?

In Taoist traditions, the three levels of consciousness of Jing, Qi, and Shen are referred to as the Three Treasures. In Vedic lineage they are named Vata, Pitta, and Kapha. In most Christian-based ideologies, the Father, Son, and Holy Ghost form the Trinity.

Shamans speak of the lower world, upper world, and middle world. Many wisdom modalities have belief structures with three levels of being.

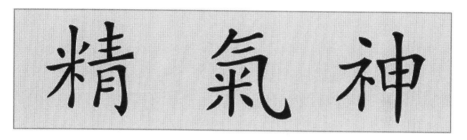

Although the names (words) are different, the finish line where the names (words) direct our mind is the same. Words direct our mind in a general direction of thought, however, it is rarely the word that adequately paints the picture. Words are limited in ability to describe, often just getting us in the ball park of where the word is attempting to point our mind. There is a Taoist saying, "The finger that points at the moon is not the moon. Look to where the finger points."

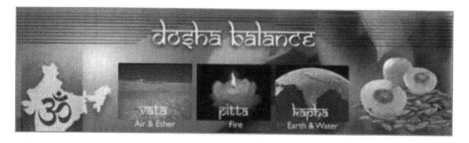

These three levels point to a solid, liquid, and gas. Keep in mind that a solid still has more space than matter.

> *Solids*—Jing, Kapha, the Son, the lower world.
> *Liquids*—Qi, Pitta, the Holy Ghost, the middle world.
> *Gas*—Shen, Vata, Consciousness, the Father, upper world.

Solids, liquids, and gases are all waves of light that have been frozen to the corresponding levels. The matter within these levels move according to the frequency at which they are assigned.

Within this practice, the three levels of physical, breath, and visualization are used to align the bodies.

The physical Jing alignment starts with properly stacking the joints for optimal structure support. The Qi alignment pertains to the quality and capacity of the breath. The Shen alignment relates to the visualization techniques.

> *I Qi Li* (the mind leads the Qi). These three overlay the main dan tien or focal points in TCM. One ruling the head region, one the heart, and one the low abdomen.

Looking at aligning the physical body from a standing position:

Consider that the human is placed within the Wood Element. Then consider how wood (a plant) grows. Wood grows in two opposite directions—one downward with roots seeking water, the other upward seeking sunlight. When aligning the physical body this is taken into account by extending in both directions from the core of the body. Take into mind the whole solar plexus area with the naval being the base and the heart being the top. From the naval down is the rooting action, the front of the low belly from pelvic floor to naval lifts then pulls back through the naval towards the middle of the kidney area and down into the tailbone, which drops like an anchor into the earth. This is one of three prongs that root into the earth. The other two being each foot. With the legs lightly bent, and kneecaps and feet facing forward and the tailbone dropping, one will grip the ground with the toes. The upper body action opposes this root with a light and graceful lifting of the inner self through the crown of the head.

It takes effort to root, and grace to blossom. Here we show the three: rooting, blossoming, and the center conduit object.

Jing Qi Shen
The Jing / Kapha body
The Qi / Pita body
The Shen / Vata body
Namaste of Shen

A *dosha (doṣa),* according to Ayurveda, is one of three bodily humors that make up one's constitution. These teachings are also known as the Tridosha theory.

The central concept of Ayurvedic medicine is the theory that health exists when there is a balance between three fundamental bodily humours, or doshas, called Vata, Pitta, and Kapha.

The presence of Kapha is explained to be thick, dense, mucus, sluggish, cool, solids in lower bowels, sleeps well, slow to change direction or make decision, and earth-like qualities and features. Ruling over the lower abdomen.

Kapha is the principle of protection, nourishment, and stability. It is associated with the earth element. People with a predominance of Kapha in their nature tend to have a heavier frame, think and move more leisurely, and are stable. When balanced, it creates calmness, sweetness, and loyalty. When excessive, Kapha can cause weight gain, congestion, and resistance to healthy change.

> *Kapha is the body fluid principle which relates to mucus, lubrication, and the carrier of nutrients.*
>
> —Wikipedia.

When Pita is present, the energy is of a fiery nature, warm almost hot, quick to change directions and make decisions, flame shaped, thinner edges, hot digestive systems, the heat of a digestive system from the process of changing food to waste (similar to a compost pile radiating heat). Ruling over the heart and solar plexus region.

Pitta is the principle of transformation represented in our digestion of ideas, sensory experiences, emotions, and food. It is associated with the Fire Element. People with a predominance of Pitta in their nature tend to be muscular, smart, and determined. If balanced, a Pitta is warm, intelligent, and a good leader. If out of balance, Pitta can make us critical, irritable, and aggressive.

> *Pitta is the bilious humour, or that secreted between the stomach and bowels and flowing through the liver and permeating spleen, heart, eyes, and skin; its chief quality is heat. It is the energy principle which uses bile to direct digestion and hence metabolism.*
> —Wikipedia

Vata presence shifts to a nervous energy and is most ethereal, therefore belonging to the head region (mind/shen).

Vata is the principle of movement and change. It can be identified as the Wind Element. People with a predominance of Vata in their nature tend to be thin, light, and quick in their thoughts and actions. Change is a constant part of life. When Vata is balanced, they are creative, enthusiastic, and lively. But if Vata becomes excessive, they may develop anxiety, insomnia, dry skin, or irregular digestion.

> *Vāta or Vata (wind) is the impulse principle necessary to mobilize the function of the nervous system. It affects the windy humour, flatulence, gout, rheumatism, etc.*
> —Wikipedia

Part 4

The Four Pillars

Hour	Day	Month	Year
戊	庚	丙	己
子	寅	戌	卯

Four Pillars

Divided into two parts: Pre (Before) Heaven
and Post (After) Heaven. The pillars of self.
Outside (sun) Before Heaven. Inside (moon) Before Heaven.
Outside (sun) After Heaven. Inside (moon) After Heaven.

First—your outer appearance to the world given to you by DNA—your family line. This is not just physical appearance, it is also the emotional and mental appearance you come with into this world. It is a raw essence and is mutated by your acquired knowledge and upbringing.

Second—your inner emotional ways built from the environment in which you mature and grow independence techniques formed from upbringing (parents).

Third—the method in which you approach family. Your matured self—this is often known as the "day master" reflected in your mate. After all, we tend to gravitate to those who "complete us."

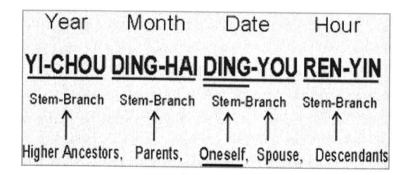

Fourth—How you approach descendants—reproduction and sexuality. How will you use it, and what blood or form will you leave behind.

Nature/Nurture

Think of yourself as a common computer. The nature (Before Heaven) of oneself is the DNA construction of the computer—what year it was built and what factory it was built in will determine the outer casing, screen, capabilities, compatibilities, size, and the software of its generation.

The nurture (After Heaven) of oneself includes the environment software, memory, browsing history, cookies, and hardware adjustments to the original item.

Part 5

Balancing the Elements

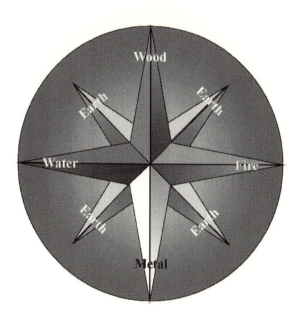

The Five Elements

What are the Five Elements?

The Five Elements could also be called the Five Activities to describe the five root energies found on planet earth. Although each of the five have qualities most visible in relation to the seasons of nature, they can be observed in all ten thousand aspects of life. All things are birthed, all things go through death—seasons, plants, people, relationships, businesses, towns, communities, and so on. The Five Elements are observed by viewing the four main seasons and the full expression of each season coming to fruition, or the five seasons if taking into account the division of the summer season into early summer and late summer. Within each season each element is also present: the first days of spring show the most sprouting (wood), the next duration of time warms (fire influence) as sprouts grow, and mid spring may express a balanced (earth) sprout with equal root and upward stalk. Moving into late spring, the culling (metal) of what will make it and what will fall away, and the last few days of spring transform (water expression) the plant up and out with the budding of flowers to come.

Start with observing what relates to the wood element in the spring season. The sprouting of plant life, the explosion of creature population through birthing of new babies, the inspiration for a new business and plans being drawn, people meeting and beginning relationships, the first members coming together for a community or town, and so on. Observe when nature begins to go from the dormant state of no growth in winter to the green of new life showing up in the spring.

The first eight years of a human's life starting from germination onward is related to the wood element, the time when a youngster would be birthed, and seeds are planted. Seeds that are supported by the surrounding environment will sprout and develop roots and a thickening stalk to support the later fruits. This of course depends on the quality of the seed derived from its ancestors as much as the quality of the environment supporting the germinating and growing seed. During this phase, observation of patterns offers the plant or youngster an intuitive knowledge of how to co-exist in the realm of life present around them.

The wood element relates to eyes and the observers housed in the liver. During the wood phase, the eyes gather information on how the world assembles in the environment around the subject. What the subject views sets the stage for future behavior. This is a collection of information time. The attributes of youth, whether in a plant, season, or person, tend to have a springy and flexible nature. Plants during this phase are more pliable, and children often show more flexibility and a bounce to their step than adults. What occurs during the springtime directly affects the results of the rest of the seasons. The wood element collects water to grow so that the fire can be nourished. Did it drought? Then the harvest could be a lighter yield. Was it an overly wet spring where many seeds were washed away or rotted? Was the moisture and heat just right, giving the seed a chance to root and be nourished properly so the plant developed correctly to bear a balanced crop? What the plant is made of during this phase will show up in all other seasons.

Once the wood roots and develops a stronger stalk with some foliage, the flowers pop open in accordance with the late spring season warming in to the early days of summer showing the blooming expression of the fire element. When a youngster has begun to blossom, we begin to see the type of person he or she will be.

With a properly supported spring season, the expression of life explodes like fire with rapid growth of whatever has been cultivated thus far. A plant goes from sprouting to bolting, a person develops from child-like form, mind and activities to young adult ways through the process of puberty. Puberty is a fire phase where an individual's movement spreads outward like a growing fire lasting from age eight to thirty-three. Their physical body bolts upward and outward. Height is established, chest expands, hair grows out of more locations, emotions teeter on explosive tendencies, the mind moves from the vast imagination of childhood to flowering of potential of dreams, and the youngster flowers into its unique self contrasting with what is around it. The fire element relates to the heart, original soul and to the tongue and tastes. One could say this is where the individual's own tastes for things and life develops and begins to express itself. Relationships blossom, businesses expand and become more noticed. Timing in blossoming is imperative for success of future elements. Should one flower to early it could risk the last frosts of spring where the blooms could be lost, resulting in a lack of ability to fruit. This could be starting a family to early (which is the fruit) and could weigh down the plant before its structure is in place to properly sustain the fruit. In a relationship it can be viewed as lust that burnt out before love grew. A business idea that is a little before its time. Fire element expressions include upward and outward movement, more visibility from the light produced so the individual can see and be seen—such as a plant flowering towards the sun so it may be seen by the bees. The joyful sounding note of G is the musical expression of fire.

The pollination from the flowering reaches the midway point of life where fruit is birthed. This is one example of the earth element. The earth element belongs in the center. It is the sweet spot so to speak. Fruiting expression of the earth element shows the work done thus far. How well the wood element rooted and grew, and the fire element exploded flowers are now seen in how well the stalk and stems hold up the developing fruit, and how well the flowering produced the proper pollen. Earth element corresponds to the middle age of one's life. During the earth phase of human relationships or businesses, the fruits of one's labor grow for later harvest during the reaping stage of the metal element. Along the way, weeding is necessary to keep the nutrients going into the fruit-bearing plant instead of scattering around into useless weeds. The earth element relates to the mouth and touch. During this time we see the individual's ability to sustain oneself through self nourishment. The family support is weaned as the individual becomes in touch with what is needed to sustain him or herself during the earth phase years of thirty-three to fifty-eight, shown both in the ability to feed and house oneself—if the development was properly grown and supported. The flip side would show the improper growth with misshapen fruits and lack of quantity. This is the middle of one's life and the most balanced expression of one's work and efforts. The balance between having one's parents care for you in the early years and the potential of one's offspring caring for them during their senior years. Thus it's a balance point when the individual has the best chance to be in a balanced state. The middle of life or earth phase relates to the note of C. Thus middle C on a piano or middle of the grand staff. Fire births earth by having consumed its fuel of wood past the point of burning embers all the way to ash. Earth meets fire as it apexes and descends from the hot of fire to the lesser heat and warming that is earth. Earth, of course, then goes from its balance point between the hotness of fire to the coolness of metal setting in. Still pliable, but it's cooling and congealing and time is ticking. The view from wood and fire that used to show endless time and bountiful opportunities of open doors becomes the realization that the midway point of that life expression is now in process and approaching rapidly. This is the time when a living thing has established its foundation, built its walls, provided a roof and filled a nest with feathers along with gathering life-sustaining items of water and nourishment.

Cutting away fruit by the cool weather of fall creeping in or the bladed strike of a machete happens either way. This is the first time the energy begins to wain. Our life-force energy begins to dwindle, the body begins its decent from birth and balanced state of all three levels of self. Friends and family begin to pass, and businesses begin transforming the fruits into a new business venture or nest egg. Metal represents the moving or removal of the bulk of life, the setting sun at the end of a long day or life's work. Occurring from ages fifty-eight to eighty-three, the view of the story of one's life has thickened and congeals as it heads into its first cool season. As burning hot embers of a fire collapse losing their flair and flame into the warm ashes of earth, the remains cool to metal or minerals from the initial wood's physical make up. As the ash is compressed into various elemental groupings, the type of metal forms—meaning, what kind of metal will it become, and the best metals withstand high temperatures. The metal element is reflected in the fall, lungs, the setting sun, skin, large intestine, nose, po shen, body hair, by the color white, integrity and benevolence vs. grief, sorrow, sadness, and loneliness. Musically it relates to the cutting sound of the D note. Metal is the result of cooling and hardening earth, and feeds the transformational water process of melting the mineral content of the metal to transport into the new wood plant or expression. Here the harvest is collected. Reaping from the sowing of one's seed, caring for the flowering stage, and having borne fruit. The quality of this season is largely dependent on the life expression's ability thus far and of the environment in which it was cultivated. What varieties and qualities the harvest yields comes from the farmer's (in this case the inner consciousness's) actions thus far. The consciousness's efforts driving the entity's life becomes solid. The expression is fixed and in place, not that small changes can or cannot be made, just that the large structure is set. This harvest is what one will have to work with. On a lifelong level this would mean the body is set, not much more changes. The mind has its lifelong interests and ways expressed and set. Much would need to occur to make large changes. The ways of dealing with emotions and the understanding of qi is clearly evident in one's life arena. The life of a relationship is solid and reflecting if it will transform and infinitely divide into a new expression of its root self, or die off to begin a new type of root elsewhere. It's as if the future self reveals itself in one's mirrored reflection. Metal element carries similarity to the air element of some traditions. The air is simply the mineral of oxygen, and one could place this easily in the metal category. Oxygen is a space holder, the amount of oxygen determines the metal's state.

Water transforms or washes away. Either way it will give birth to a new wood expression—babies of life. It is the building block or foundation of the universe. Water is delivered to the space in rocks that hold the potential for life. Because it belongs to the reproductive organs, one could relate it to the womb. The holding space of all potential that can create life when an egg is able to be watered by semen. When these two meet, the wood or seed of life may begin to grow. The new life will be a product of the infinite divisibility of two to create the one. The transformation process takes the nourishing minerals of metal and transports them to wood through a filtering process. The wood's future depends on the quality of the water or ancestral DNA including its mineral (metal) content. Water shows the unfathomable depth potential of life. The deep sound of the note A even in the higher registers may almost resinate in the bones. It is the coldest—at times so cold it burns—of the elemental expressions relating to the winter of one's life.

The previous seasons will culminate during this phase. How one survives during the winter years will be mostly from the cultivation of one's seeds. What community and family are around, what choices one may have made as one's life span draws to its conclusion during ages eight-three to 108—letting go is the inevitable theme. Letting go is a charged word that can imply loss. The wisdom view of this time's highest expression would see it as giving back—feeding itself back into the new rooting plant of its time through sharing of wisdom, resources, and medicines collected from the duration of the journey thus far.

In a plant's life this would show what the use of the plant became. The harvest took the fruit off the crop and it is now being used in a kitchen at best, or recycled in a compost heap. Harvested fruits highest potential is to be used or properly saved for future use. Maybe it is being served with tonight's dinner or preserved as jam. The action of transformation includes the turning of base materials into a new material. Water expresses in cold, salty, midnight blue, hidden danger and potential, ears, kidneys, bones, bladder, ancestral energies, DNA, endocrine system, brain, reproductive organs, fear, and will power.

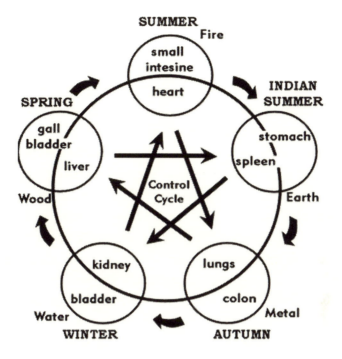

Five Elemental Body Types

Wood Head = Vertical Rectangle

Fire Head = Flame Shape

Earth Head = Square with Wide Jaw

Metal Head = High Cheek Bones

Water Head = Round in Shape

Lessons from Gardening:

When a seed is planted it requires a certain amount of heat (campfire heat) to germinate and almost no light (Qi illumination—such as lightning from heaven). Of course during this time it requires proper amounts of water, earth, and minerals (metals) to germinate and begin growing. This is similar to a human fetus in the womb, which resides in total darkness, yet requires the heat from the mother's body to grow. If the mother's body is too cold (or too hot for that matter) the imbalance presses upon the fetus and ailments may arrive. Each growing item in the sphere of the earth belongs to the wood element. Each piece of the wood element requires a specific environment with a correct balance of the Five Elements to thrive. The water that wets and nourishes the wood must include the proper minerals (metals) for that type of wood to flourish. The metals that are transported into the wood via the water will influence the type of wood it will become and how it will withstand Mother Nature's influences. The minerals (metals) inside the wood will also influence the fire action coming out of the wood when burned. If the wood includes many heavy minerals (metals) it tends to burn slower vs. a wood with little heavy mineral (metal) content. Also the quickness in which the wood burns will also be influenced by the amount of water residing in the wood.

Now once the seed has germinated in the proper heat temperature (first fire) and breaks through the topsoil it begins to receive nourishment from the second fire—light from the sun (real or artificial)—in order to grow. The heat temperature still applies—too cold or hot and the plant struggles to survive—however, without the second fire or light from the sun it will not grow.

Five Elements Relating to Your Practice and Life

The Five Element Theory helps you understand how natural changes within your body and outside environment affect your health. Implement the theory for your body health through the use of healing sounds. Healing Sounds are a method of displacing old stagnant prana or qi using a reverberation of sound, physical movement, and visualization. Inhalations restore fresh vibrant prana or energy to the elemental structure or organ. The exhalation purges emotion and the darkest of the element's color. The inhalation pulls in the lightest of the element's color and enhances virtues.

Healing Sounds:

木 Wood
Liver & Gall Bladder
Sound: Shiiii
Emotion: Anger
Virtue: Justice

火 Fire
Heart & Small Intestine
Sound: Haaaa
Emotion: Shock
Virtue: Courage / Respect

土 Earth
Spleen & Stomach
Sound: Whoooo
Emotion: Worry
Virtue: Knowledge

金 Metal
Lung & Large Intestine
Sound: Hissss
Emotion: Grief
Virtue: Benevolence

水 Water
Kidney & Bladder
Sound: Cheuuuu
Emotion: Fear
Virtue: Truthfulness / Sincerity

The following five protocols are references for harmonizing the body's elemental self. Detailed explanations are provided in the Zen Yoga course.

Zen Yoga: Theory, Postures, and Remedies

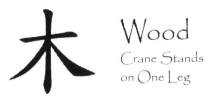

Wood
Crane Stands on One Leg

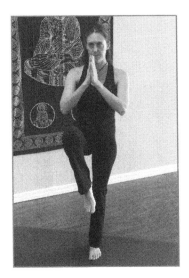

Wood—sight, **balancing**, flexibility, ages 0–8, observation.

The wood element rises to heaven and the roots reach for the center of the earth as seen in "Crane Stands on One Leg." This is also known as Tree Pose. The main emphasis is to root the foot and lift the head. Be sure to lift the head and relax the shoulders. Pay close attention to all of the toes rooting into the earth.

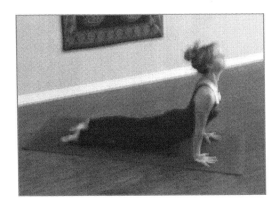

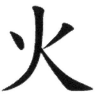

Fire
Back Bend

Fire—taste, **heart openers**, cardio, ages 8–33, speech.

The fire element expands, opens and releases energy and corresponds to back bends. The back bend is used in many yoga positions. Be sure to lift the chin and open the chest. This position is very effective in opening the Conception Vessel running down the center of the chest.

Part 5: Balancing the Elements

Earth—touch, **hips & core**, strength, ages 33–58, diet.

The earth element emulates the horizon reaching across and sinking down and corresponds to Triangle and Boat Pose. A strong emphasis should be put on distributing your weight equally on both feet. Keep your knees straight but not locked.

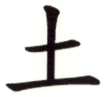

Earth
Triangle Pose

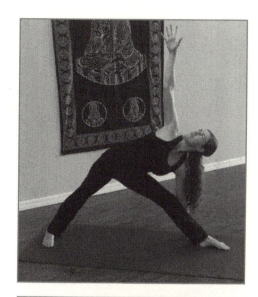

Boat Pose

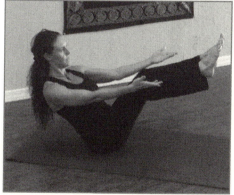

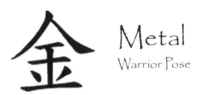 Metal
Warrior Pose

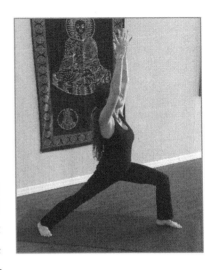

Metal—scents, **alignment**, breath, ages 58–83, air quality.

The metal element embodies a splitting energy. The weight is splitting forward distributing more weight on the front leg than on the back leg. The positioning of the front knee is very important. Do not allow the knee to move forward past the toes. Be sure to spiral the back thigh inward. Lock the rear leg and press the heel into the earth.

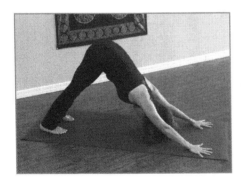

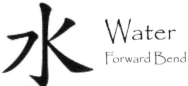 Water
Forward Bend

Water—sounds, **forward bends**, meditation/nidra, ages 83–108.

The forward bend is very much like a wave rising up and gathering its power as it draws in—therefore, it corresponds to water. The posture is excellent for opening up the Governing Vessel that runs up the center of the back.

Bringing in this level of understanding to your daily life and yoga practice occurs by considering your environment. You are what you repetitively see, say, eat/touch, breathe, and hear. All of these are vibrations—and your body will autotune to match the vibration frequencies around you. We are best served by first observing what is repetitive. Examples:

Wood

Sight Observation—What do you see every day? What images are you placing in your mind? Are you doing it consciously or is it unconsciously being done to you?

Consciously—Do you choose to watch visually stimulating shows that uplift? Or maybe your choice of images are of a downward energy including death, violence, scarcity, depression, and disfunction?

Unconsciously—What do you see as you move through your daily routine? Do you pass billboards showing that drinking and partying equal sexy women? Do you drive a road filled with fast food establishments leaving you craving a Big Mac? Do you pass banks that make you worry about your account balance?

Fire

Speech Observation—What speech do you use on an ongoing basis? Consider both internal dialogue and what actually rolls off your tongue. Is your speech truthful and compassionate (satya) or is it skewed versions of truth and harmful?

Consciously—Do you take care to stick as close to the truth as possible while attempting to be kind and considerate of others? Do you try to speak of higher and evolved conversations?

Unconsciously—Are you a broken record repeating (or thinking) what you usually say? Is this appropriate for the time and company? Are you simply parroting what your parents said without discerning if it is truth? Are you prone to gossip? When things are tough do you seek someone to commiserate with? Or someone who will try to show you the silver lining?

Earth

Diet/Texture Observation—What foods do you put in your mouth? Are they medicine or poison? Are they consciously put in to build the physical body? Or are they put in to appease the emotional self? What textures do you come across? Are they soft, warm, and inviting? Or cold, hard, and unwelcoming?

Consciously—Understanding that food is either medicine or poison. This is a moving target. For the most part we only need food to enter the body that will properly build the structure of the body. SOMETIMES we need a small dose of comfort food to heal sickness. Textures in your space—are they clean and inviting?

Unconsciously—Eating without thought. No consideration for what the body's machine needs to run optimally, thus eating based on emotion or convenience. Textures unkept, torn, dirty, harsh, or too sterile?

Metal

Air & Breath Quality—What is the general makeup of the air you breathe? Is it deep and calming? Or shallow and taxing? Do you work in the perfume department at Macy's? A toxic paint factory? Do you spend time in nature away from the city's pollutants?

Consciously—Do you take the time to breathe in deep and allow full exhalations? Are you an overactive person and do you take "breathers" throughout the day? Or are you sedentary and never get the breath "going"? Do you place clean and pleasing aromas in your home, car and office? Are you intentionally placing your self in nature?

Unconsciously—Do you jog next to a busy road? Have the windows rolled down in stagnant rush hour traffic? Place yourself in others' space who pollute the air? Park by dumpsters or live near landfills and airports?

Water

Sound Quality—What do you listen to daily? What do you hear that you are not listening to? Are the sounds in your environment pleasing, calming, natural, and uplifting? Do you have a perpetually screaming boss? Endless traffic? Do you hear birds, bees, wind and water? What are the people around you saying? (Saying and hearing—that fire and water relationship again.) Do you listen to music that cultivates understanding, compassion, and evoking the higher self? Or is it music that speaks of who did who wrong, killing others, and the facade of partying being the route of happiness?

Consciously—Choosing to surround yourself with evolved people who will speak well around you. Keeping yourself mostly removed from your own and other's "stories" of strife and troubles. These are OK on rare occasions—everyone needs a sounding board. But is this the norm? What about the places you frequent? Are the sounds sharp, heavy, and harmful?

Unconsciously—Do you listen to daytime talk shows about people misbehaving (unconsciously giving you permission to misbehave), talk show pundits, or music that encourages the lowest of human attributes?

Take the time to observe these elements in your life. Consider where you might upgrade aspects of your life. For those of you teaching—consider these things as you set the space for your class. Do you encourage the students to enter quietly? To leave their story at the door? Is the music pleasing and of correct tone? How are the smells, lighting, cleanliness of surfaces? Does your speech and volume match the energy you want to convey?

Five Element Theory helps you understand how natural changes within your body and the outside environment affect your health. To predict and understand these dynamic changes, ancient doctors studied nature to determine what universal principles existed that could be applied to health and well-being. The Five Element Theory is what they came up with.

The five elements are Wood, Fire, Earth, Metal, and Water. They were selected based on the observations of ancient Eastern philosophers who observed that everything in the natural world embodied these elemental characteristics. Oriental Medicine uses the five elements in a time-tested, diagnostic model to analyze how the various parts of a person's body and mind interact to affect health.

The Generating Cycle

Based on the Five Element Theory, each elemental force generates or creates the next element in a sequence illustrated below:

Water generates wood. (Rain nourishes a tree.)

Wood generates fire. (Burning wood generates fire.)

Fire generates earth. (Ash is created from the fire.)

Earth generates metal. (Metal is mined from the earth.)

Metal generates water. (Water condenses on metal.)

Part 5: Balancing the Elements

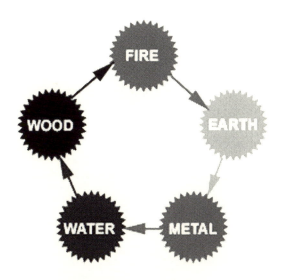

Generating (Sheng) Cycle

When applying this "supportive relationship" to the human body, we see that each internal organ embodies the energetic qualities of the element associated with it. Each organ is responsible for providing the energy needed by the next organ in the generative cycle:

Kidney (water element) supports the liver (wood element).

Liver (wood element) supports the heart (fire element).

Heart (fire element) supports the spleen (earth element).

Spleen (earth element) supports the lungs (metal element).

Lungs (metal element) support the kidneys (water element).

The Controlling Cycle

Based on the Five Element Theory, each elemental force is also associated with another element that is responsible for controlling or regulating (see below illustration):

Water controls fire. (Water puts out fire.)

Wood controls earth. (Tree roots hold clods of earth.)

Fire controls metal. (Fire can melt metal.)

Earth controls water. (A pond holds water.)

Metal controls wood. (An ax cuts wood.)

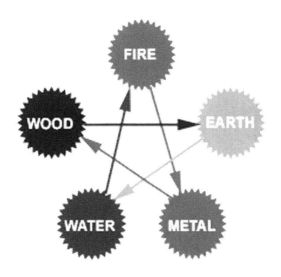

Control (Ke) Cycle

When applying this "controlling relationship" to the human body, we see that each internal organ embodies the energetic qualities of the element related to it. Each organ is responsible for providing the energy needed to keep the opposite energy in check. For example:

Kidney (water element) controls the heart (fire element).
Heart (fire element) controls the lung (metal element).
Lungs (metal element) control the liver (wood element).
Liver (wood element) controls the spleen (earth element).
Spleen (earth element) controls the kidneys (water element).

Advanced Five Element Regulation Protocols

The five elements may be seen within any living expression. There is always the sprouting, flowering, fruiting, harvesting, and returning or transforming aspects. Looking at this during one's lifespan helps to determine the natural energetic flow occurring as to best coexist with the season of your life and activities that align for that time period. Each period always begins with Wood, actually wood of wood, then moves on to fire of wood, earth of wood then metal of wood and so forth. As the season begins, it is at its newest state—thus wood of any season (say the first 15 or so days of spring, still chilly yet warmth is sprouting). As the season progresses, or opens up, you have fire of any season. Once the season matures and balances out (say midway from spring to summer) the earth element of the season expresses. This is the early decline of the season (say later in spring when the temps are warming, but not yet hot). Lastly, the water expression of any season washes away the previous season and transforms the energy toward the next season (the last days of spring, end of the school year, for example).

Use the following chart to find your current season and gain insight on coexisting.

Part 5: Balancing the Elements

WOOD Spring 木 0-8	FIRE Early Summer 火 8-33	EARTH Late Summer 土 33-58	METAL Fall 金 58-83	WATER Winter 水 83-108
WOOD Spring 木 0-8	木 0 火 土 金 水 birth	木 8 火 9 土 10 金 11 水 12	木 33 火 34 土 35 金 36 水 37	木 58 火 59 土 60 金 61 水 62	木 83 火 84 土 85 金 86 水 87
FIRE Early Summer 火 8-33	木 birth 火 土 金 水 2	木 13 火 14 土 15 金 16 水 17	木 38 火 39 土 40 金 41 水 42	木 63 火 64 土 65 金 66 水 67	木 88 火 89 土 90 金 91 水 92
EARTH Late Summer 土 33-58	木 2 火 土 金 水 4	木 18 火 19 土 20 金 21 水 22	木 43 火 44 土 45 金 46 水 47	木 68 火 69 土 70 金 71 水 72	木 93 火 94 土 95 金 96 水 97
METAL Fall 金 58-83	木 4 火 土 金 水 6	木 23 火 24 土 25 金 26 水 27	木 48 火 49 土 50 金 51 水 52	木 73 火 74 土 75 金 76 水 77	木 98 火 99 土 100 金 101 水 102
WATER Winter 水 83-108	木 6 火 土 金 水 8	木 28 火 29 土 30 金 31 水 32	木 53 火 54 土 55 金 56 水 57	木 78 火 79 土 80 金 81 水 82	木 103 火 104 土 105 金 106 水 107

© 2012 Zen Wellness All rights reserved

Zen Yoga: Theory, Postures, and Remedies

Wood Protocols	Seated Practice	Standing Practice	Moving Practice
Beginner Jing	Tongue Wood Point	Side Kick stretch stretching abductors	Wood Healing Sound
Beginner Qi	Horary Acupressure: GB41 LR1	Stand like a Tree	Wood Animal Healing Deer
Beginner Shen	1-10	Liver – Gallbladder Meridian Breathing	Liver Regulating
Intermediate Jing	Shaking the Heavenly Pillar	Immortal Straightens Beard	Tiger Wags Tail
Intermediate Qi	Acute Acupressure: GB1	8 Vessel Crescent Moon	Qi Breathing: Holding Inhale
Intermediate Shen	Projection (future season)	Leading Qi: Linking Vessels	Striking the Bag
Advanced Jing	Mudra: Sun & Moon	Sleeping Position	Extend the Waist
Advanced Qi	Regulating Acupressure: + GB43 LV8 / - GB38 LV2	Dragon Stretches Claws	Tapping: Liver & Gallbladder Meridian
Advanced Shen	Mantra: OM	Iron Body	Qi Emission: Liver

Fire Protocols	Seated Practice	Standing Practice	Moving Practice
Beginner Jing	Tongue Fire Point	Hold the Moon on Golden Plate	Fire Healing Sound
Beginner Qi	Horary Acupressure: SI5 HT8 TW6 PC8	Embrace the Heart	Fire Animal Healing Hawk
Beginner Shen	Dragon Hides & Tiger Leaps	SI, HT, TW, PC Meridian Breathing	Heart Regulating
Intermediate Jing	Raising Arms	Monkey lifts a cauldron	Buddha Palm
Intermediate Qi	Acute Acupressure: SI19 TW23	8 Vessel Ba push two poles	Qi Breathing: Longer Exhale
Intermediate Shen	Pao Yi	Leading Qi: Govern & Concept Vessels	Old Man Searches
Advanced Jing	Mudra: Namaste	Cobra Rise	Swallow Returns to Nest
Advanced Qi	Regulating Acupress: + SI3 HT9 TW3 PC8 / - SI8 HT7 TW10 PC7	Taoist Horse	Tapping: HT, SI, TW, PC
Advanced Shen	Mantra: Harr	Iron Body	Qi Emission: Heart

Earth Protocols	Seated Practice	Standing Practice	Moving Practice
Beginner Jing	Tongue Earth Point	Baby Dancer Pose	Earth Healing Sound
Beginner Qi	Horary Acupressure: ST36 SP3	Stand firm on earth	Earth Animal Healing Monkey
Beginner Shen	5 Element Fusion	Stomach & Spleen Meridian Breathing	Stomach Regulating
Intermediate Jing	Twisting to both sides	Side Po	Butterfly Dive
Intermediate Qi	Acute Acupressure: ST1	8 Vessel Twist body like rope	Qi Breathing: Equal
Intermediate Shen	Ren Wu Zhong	Leading Qi: Belt Vessel	Turtle Breathing
Advanced Jing	Mudra: Stomach mudra (Pachan Mudra	Boat pose	Monkey Dances on Clouds
Advanced Qi	Regulating Acupress: + ST41 SP2 / - ST45 SP5	Inverted T stance	Tapping: Stomach & Spleen meridian
Advanced Shen	Mantra: Om Mani Padme Hum	Iron Body	Qi Emission: Spleen

Metal Protocols	Seated Practice	Standing Practice	Moving Practice
Beginner Jing	Tongue Metal Point	Half-way Lift	Metal Healing Sound
Beginner Qi	Horary Acupressure: LI11 LU8	Hold Golden Qi Ball	Metal Animal Healing Tiger
Beginner Shen	Cutting away the pain	Lung & Lg. Intestine Meridian Breathing	Lung Regulating
Intermediate Jing	Seated half way lift	One Foot Treads the Sky	Natural Palm
Intermediate Qi	Acute Acupressure: LI20	Santi	Qi Breathing: Longer inhalation
Intermediate Shen	Reflection (past season)	Leading Qi: Thrusting Vessel	Dry Crying
Advanced Jing	Mudra: Metal (Chin Maya)	Plank (high & low)	Splitting Clouds
Advanced Qi	Regulating Acupress: + LI11 LU9 / - LI2 LU5	Crane to 7 star	Tapping: Lung & Lg. Intest meridians
Advanced Shen	Mantra: Flute Sounds	Iron Body	Qi Emission: Lung

Zen Yoga: Theory, Postures, and Remedies

Water Protocols	Seated Practice	Standing Practice	Moving Practice
Beginner Jing	Tongue Water Point	Four Fingers Press Earth	Water Healing Sound
Beginner Qi	Horary Acupressure: BL66 KD10	Stand in River	Water Animal Healing Bear
Beginner Shen	Red Dragon	Bladder & Kidney Meridian Breathing	Kidney Regulating
Intermediate Jing	Kidney Rubbing	Forward bend holding back of Calves	Cat gazes at Moon
Intermediate Qi	Acute Acupressure: BL1 & BL2	Bow / Ride Tiger	Qi Breathing: Holding Exhale
Intermediate Shen	Keeping Still	Leading Qi: Heel Vessel	Dredging
Advanced Jing	Mudra: Infinity	Down Dog/ Cat Stretch	Pushing Elbow in Goose Stance
Advanced Qi	Regulating Acupress: + BL67 KD7/-BL65 KD1	Seven Star Stance (press earth)	Tapping: Bladder & KD meridians
Advanced Shen	Mantra: Reem	Iron Body	Qi Emission: Kidney

Part 6

Prana/Qi
The Sixth Element

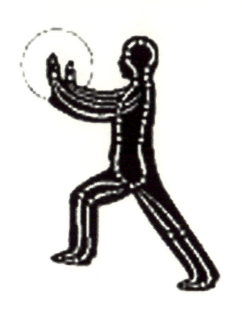

The Sixth Element—Prana (Qi)

The theory of the Five Elements is the base of form. The sixth element—prana—is an almost intangible element that gives movement to form. There are two types of movement from form (yin and yang, of course). There is movement that comes from within form and expresses outward, and there is movement that comes from outside of form and acts upon form.

The external movement is an influence of nature, gravity, or creature, such as rain loosing soil around rocks and creating an avalanche. Internal movement derives from an inward dwelling consciousness that inspires the object to move. Objects that have an indwelling consciousness belong to the wood element and are moved by prana or qi allowing the wood element to stir and or move—such as a plant turning towards the sun, or a deer moving to water.

Prana is able to be sensed—thus the sixth sense. It's an intuitive knowing, such as being able to tell that a space one just entered has a "good" or "bad" vibe. As all Five Elements belong to a sense organ, the sixth element—prana—belongs to intuition or a deep knowing. Maybe where the saying "trust your gut" comes from? In earlier years, speaking of prana could land you in the loony bin or burned at the stake. Nowadays, we have sophisticated cameras that can image our auric fields and heat-seeking infrared technology that is able to find body heat (prana), giving us hard evidence of the prana within. The flow of prana within a plant or creature is in direct relation to the health and vitality of the organism. A yogi is able to direct prana to achieve asanas (postures) and deliberately enhance his or her well-being. Prana moves through nadis or meridians and may be accessed through specific areas called Marma points (or acupuncture points). These points are arranged with the Five Element structure to create homeostasis in the energy field from application of how the prana is generated or controlled.

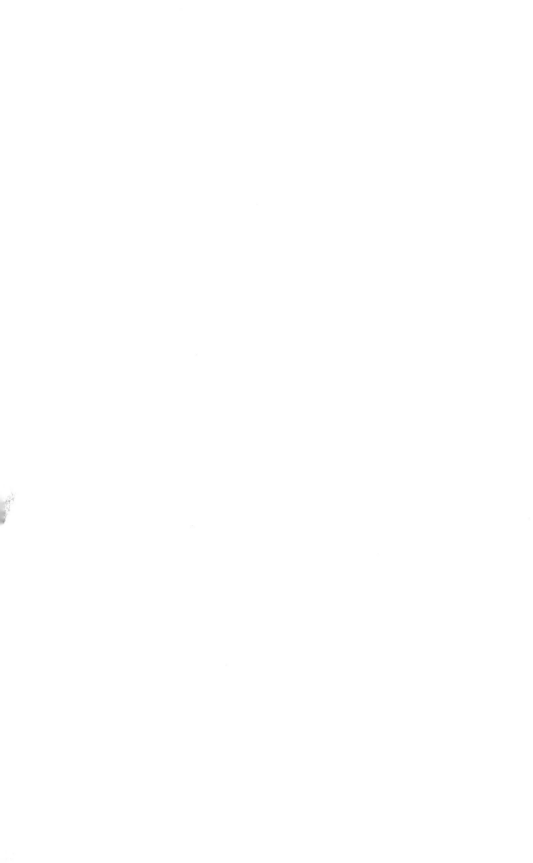

Part 7
The Seven Chakras

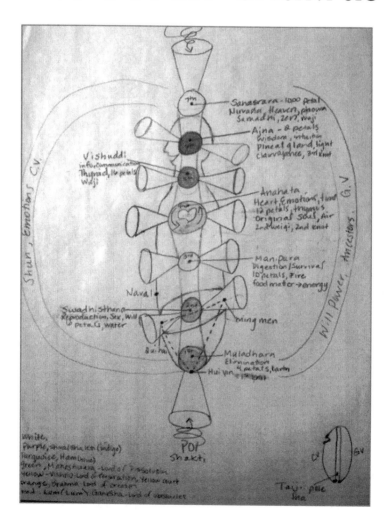

What Are the Seven Chakras?

The Seven Chakras are seen in many wisdom traditions. Expressed in the seven heavens, the seven dimensions, seven colors of the light spectrum seen in the rainbow (Roy G. Biv).

Each tradition uses seven to attempt to explain the solidifying of light. Red being the heaviest of colors and violet being the lightest with the other colors as in-between phases of the thickening light. Some traditions speak of how the Seven Chakras are actually the Five Elements bookended by one gate to the earth and one gate to the heavens. On planet earth creatures reside in these seven dimensions (well six dimensions—we can only view the seventh, not reside in it). However, there are infinite levels of dimensions in the universe. We simply reside in the seven belonging to the earthly realm. The chakras run vertically parallel to the spine through the central part of the torso, neck, and head. Stacking on top of each other as spinning wheels of light located within an energetic structure or channel sometimes called the Tai Ji Pole or Sushumna-nadi that runs from the perineum to the bahui point at the crown of the head. The wheels of light are centrally located within the body in this channel and connect to the front of the body and back of the body through vortex-like tunnels. The tunnels of chakras 2–6 connected to the front of the body relate to the future, shun, emotions, and Conception Vessel. The connection of tunnels for chakras 2–6 on the back of the body are associated with the past, ancestors, and the will power one arrived with on this plane, as well as the Governing Vessel. Yet another expression of the root and crown chakras being gates to heaven and earth. The Governing and Conception vessels connect at the root and crown.

Where do they reside in the body?

The red root Muladhara chakra found at the base of the torso of a creature rests at the perineum near the base of the spine and is drawn with four petals. The root chakra is all about basic elimination of form. How the elimination process is working is the root expression of the life form's ability to sustain itself. It is said to express the connection to the earth, physical survival, general health, root, source, support, vital part, the heaviest element of earth, "I live" Po, the Ganesha (Lord of obstacles), and the sound of LAM. The ultimate feminine point of the chakras. This chakra directly relates to form. Form exiting the body either by stool, urine, or birth. It relates to the feminine or yin by its clouded or thick nature. Example of urine that was clear drinking water now clouded with waste leaving the body. It went in clear, or yang, and left turbid or yin. It is all about grounding or rooting into the earth. This chakra can be described as the gate to earth. The quality of this chakra will be the foundation of how the other chakras are stabilized. Because it will determine how well a creature feels at home and is supported so the other areas of its life have a container from which to grow. Thus it's the base dimension of our earthly experience, described like a dot, such as on a map, showing where one is, the root or location. We are able to ascertain where one is in life by their root chakra. What are they connected to? What environment are they rooted in? The one point of connection.

One step up from the root or base chakra is the second chakra Swadhisthana—colored as orange, the second heaviest color of our earthly light spectrum, the sound of VAM, "I Feel," and drawn with six petals, second heaviest element of water connected to Brahma (Lord of Creation). A glowing expression of one's sexuality, pleasures and desires. Residing inside the hara of the body or dan tien (brass basin) it relates to the powerhouse or battery of the energy body and in some traditions to the element of water, which also corresponds to sexuality and reproductive organs. This is one of two chakras that rest on a diagonal plane connecting the mingmen and qi hai points of the basin. The first split, coming from the one centered root point at the foundation of the brass basin to create a viewpoint of the rim of the basin. This level or dimension is viewed as a flat line. No longer simply a dot, now a line with two opposing directions. Flat to express the two-dimensional view. Simply yin and yang if you will, not yet expressing depth, only distance. The one has jumped a dimension and became the two—or, on a descending view, the two dropping into becoming one.

The third chakra up known as Manipura is colored as yellow and drawn with ten petals, associated with the sound of RAM, and "I do." It's the third heaviest element of fire, and the third dimension of form or 3D. When the flat line of the second gains depth, it shows size such as a wave differing from a particle, thus giving a 3D view. A particle shows where. A wave will not say where, but instead how big. The third heaviest color connected to the yellow court and Vishnu (Lord of preservation). Located between the navel and chest at the solar plexus near the stomach, spleen, and pancreas which also relate to the color of yellow. In the Taoist tradition the yellow court is where much of the work is needed to be done, appropriately named the yellow court for the king's place of unfinished business—akin to nourishment from ingestion of food waiting to be assimilated into the body in the holding container that is the stomach. It's a place of personal power and emotions. Also within Taoist alchemy the work in the yellow court deals with all unfinished business and old emotions for a pure ascent upwards or at the closing of one's experience of this go around in form. If the emotions are left unprocessed they may cloud the soul while exiting the body and compel or repel the soul back into form to complete the still unresolved issues. The practice to care for this is known as "Illumination of the Golden Court" or "Golden Flower." The chakra in the center of the earthly line of chakras is located at the heart center or center of the chest. This is where the three earthly chakras and the three heavenly chakras mix. Expressed by the color green such as the wood element in Taoist traditions and as air in the Ayurvedic traditions. The wood element is comprised of blue heaven and yellow earth. Wood element belongs to humans, creatures, and plants. Taught as, "Man divides heaven and earth."

The fourth chakra moves from simply expressing the depth of the wave at the third chakra or dimension to now showing the movement of the wave. It is the flow of time or "e"-motion in the fourth dimension. It represents that which is in motion, what has passed, and that which is anticipated to come that stirs the heart and original soul. Emotions color the view of the soul here. When the emotions are calm like a placid lake, then the soul receives the least distorted view, otherwise heavy emotional movement shades the soul's view in direct relation to the strength and nature of the emotion. Drawn with twelve petals, gives the sound of YAM, associated with Maheshwara (Lord of dissolution), "I love," and also named Anahata. Ultimately, this chakra expresses pure compassion unconditional love, forgiveness, and tolerance. Alchemy of turning into the precious jade stone or emerald city of Oz where the original soul resides, including the actual heart organ known as the most important organ or Emperor organ.

Vishuddha, "the fifth chakra" or the throat chakra, is located at the base of the neck/throat. Drawn with sixteen petals to express the more dynamic expression of the earthly dimensions. Expressed with the sound HAM, the color blue of the fifth chakra is now reflecting heaven energies (top three chakras) instead of earth energies (lowest three chakras). Also related to the mastering of speech and clear communication, affirmation of "I express." Here the information resting in the throat chakra exchanges with the heart chakra's timing for fortune. The throat chakra is to speak satya (truth) for peak performance. Associated with the thyroid.

Ajna, the "sixth chakra," is drawn with two petals and is located at the center of the forehead between the brows as the "third eye" center. Expressed with the sound of OM, the color violet, and "I see." The information obtained at the fifth chakra and mixed with the timing element of the fourth chakra expresses in the sixth chakra as wisdom, building one's intuition. Governing incoming and outgoing thoughts taking us out of physical horizontal reality (Fibonacci curve) into divinity or vertical reality (binary curve). The third eye is an expression of what once was or could be obtained. Depicted in Egyptian times as the basis of the great pyramid. In the great pyramid, there lies a chamber where the heavenly spiral of qi descends and the upward spiral of earth qi meets. When one lays down with this chakra aligned, it is said to open the third eye. The Anja chakra is honored by placing a bindi to worship one's intellect, and thus ensure our thoughts, speech, actions, habits, and, ultimately, pure soul are increased by concentration and respecting the namaste within. A balanced sixth chakra reflects a balanced mind. Right and left brain working evenly together and with the ability to easily access both or switch between as desired. Not being pulled by one side or the other.

Sahasrara the "seventh" or crown chakra is drawn with one thousand petals and is located just above the top of the head. Expressed with the absence of sound, colored white, and "I am." Connected to the divine and our higher selves. The place that removes the separation of self from everything else. Depicted in wisdom traditions by a halo of sorts. This chakra is said to be unreachable while in the physical body, yet can be seen when looking up. The feather on the head of a Native American, the turban of a Hindi Indian, the topknot of a Taoist monk all serve as conduits to occupy the seventh chakra so the energy may flow down into the earthly energetic body. This chakra supplies prana to the pineal gland.

What are the common imbalances and symptoms?

First Chakra

Chronic low back pain, sciatica, varicose veins, constipation, rectal tumors, cancer, violent outbursts, knee problems, testicular cancer, hemorrhoids, inability to provide for oneself.

Second Chakra

Gynecological problems, pelvic/lower back pain, sexual potency, kidney, ovarian, uterine and urinary problems. Inability to differentiate one's own feelings from others. Lack of self worth, martyr complex. Blame, guilt, and money issues.

Third Chakra

Arthritis, gastric ulcers, intestine issues, pancreatitis/diabetes, indigestion, chronic or acute anorexia and bulimia, liver dysfunction, hepatitis, adrenal dysfunction. Poor health, depression, no motivation or follow through, waves of anger, rage, fear, greed, jealousy, judgement and criticism. Inability to manifest, and sometimes destroy. Metabolic disorders. Lack of self esteem, confidence and self-respect, distrust of others.

Fourth Chakra

Mitral valve prolapse, cardiomegaly, asthma/allergy, lung cancer, bronchial pneumonia, upper back, shoulder, breast cancer. Resentment, fear, bitterness, decrease in love of life. Insincerity, insecurity, isolation.

Fifth Chakra

Raspy throat, chronic sore throats, stiff neck, mouth ulcers, gum issues, temporomandibular joint issues, scoliosis, laryngitis, swollen glands, thyroid issues. Lack of personal expression, not following one's dreams, lack of personal manifestation power. Blocking internal organs' energy release through throat. Liver fire stagnating and creating phlegm known as "Plum Pit Qi." Refusal to communicate or silence for control and attention. Suppression of pain, depression, anger or violence. Lack of creativity.

Sixth Chakra

Brain tumors, hemorrhage, stroke, neurological disturbances, blindness, deafness, full spinal difficulties, learning disabilities, seizures, fear of self-evaluation, dulled intuition, misuse of intellect, repeating life lessons without learning. Arrogance. Firm views and opinions that cannot be moved around. Over-rationalization vs. experience. Rigid belief structors in relation to creation. Static and misinterpretation of events. Nightmares and delusion.

Seventh Chakra

Paralysis, genetic disorders, bone cancer and bone problems, MS, and ALS. Distrust of life, lack of faith or belief, basic distrust of life, attitudes, values, ethics, and courage. Lack of meaning in life or purpose of direction. Confusion, apathy, boredom, depression.

Balancing Chakras on the Jing Qi Shen Level

Jing, Qi, Shen and the Seven Chakras

Chakras reside on a qi level. However, they are affected by the state of the physical and/or shen bodies. If the movement of blood in the physical body is sluggish, then its stagnation impacts the qi and shen bodies. If the shen body is disturbed, the qi body is depleted to compensate. Then, of course, if the qi level of the chakras are off, they disturb both the physical and shen levels. As each chakra resides in a vital area of the physical body, they each naturally affect that which is around them, so balancing chakras is done across the board through all three bodies. Each region is best kept physically pliable and firm, and are served by visual relaxation techniques for each region. Managing chakras is not only done horizontally and locally to stabilize a certain chakra's region, but vertically as well. Meaning, the chakras below and above the imbalanced chakra are also managed. In this way the imbalanced chakra has support from below and above, creating a growth-conducive environment. Some of the methods to manage the chakras listed below are used on multiple chakras (sometimes all)—such as the Golden Qi Ball exercise, "Clearing the Seven Chakras," smudging, and 1-10 meditation. Think "Flexible body, flexible mind."

Root Chakra Balancing

Jing—hip opening, pelvic stabilization such as standing on a boat or pelvic clockwork, Kegels, lifting of the hui yin, and muladbahnda (root chakra lock) Merdain massage, movement, and tapping for bladder, kidney, spleen, stomach, liver, and gallbladder meridians.

Qi—deep breath work, building heat, sound of LAM, light therapy, rubies, garnet, red jasper, balanced diet for balanced stool. Large intestine douching with Taoist salt.

Shen—dealing with issues of safety/security in the world. Providing for one's self. Learning that one's true earthly home is the physical body—therefore, feeling at home wherever one goes (a teaching of the tortoise).

Second Chakra Balancing

Jing—core work, practice of expanding and contracting the space between the naval (qi hai) region and kidney (mingmen) region, and twists, standing on a boat and pelvic clock stabilization. Standing in a river. Meridian massage, movement, and tapping for bladder, kidney, spleen, stomach, liver, and gallbladder meridians.

Qi—deep breath work, stones of amber or citrine, balanced and safe sexual activity and good hygiene, plenty of water, building heat. Herbal formulas using ginseng and He Shu Wu. Taoist salt ingestion.

Shen—work not for the fruits of your labor, work for the sake of being able to work.

Third Chakra Balancing

Jing—Uddiyana bandha (abdominal pulling in and up under rib cage). Pressing on stomach and aortic valve. Core work. Standing on a boat. Meridian massage, movement, and tapping for bladder, kidney, spleen, stomach, liver, and gallbladder meridians. Deep resonant healing sounds for all organs.

Qi—deep breath work, tigers eye, gold, absorbing downward heat from the lower heart by fire-path breath, both of Taoist and Hatha traditions. Healing sounds are used for emotion sedation and virtue tonification. Herbal formulas using goji berries are advised, as well as other blood building agents. Maintain a balanced diet and a healthy association with food. Understand that *occasional* nourishment outside of strict diets is healthy—favorite prized foods sparingly eaten can be just the right medicine. Nourishment is not always in a salad. What you eat directly impacts the first chakra. What comes in the stomach, comes out the root chakra. Of course, the discussion of food can be viewed from the jing aspect, but here we are talking about the actions and emotions around food.

Shen—Managing trust, building self-esteem, clearing the yellow court of unresolved issues by visualizing the heat and light descending downward from the heart chakra. Build one's decision making muscle. Healing light visualization for each organ's specific coloring.

Fourth Chakra Balancing

Jing—Backbends/heart openers, shoulder work, tapping of heart, small intestine, lung, large intestine, triple warmer, and pericardium meridians. Thoracic spine opening. Adho Mukha Vrksasana.

Qi—specific pranayama, calming of the nervous system, rosemary tea, Airaide formulas, descending excess heat from heart, Taoist salt formulas.

Shen—letting go of resentments, fear and bitterness, dealing with grief and moving on, forgiveness to others and self, being nonjudgemental, practicing of giving and receiving love, stones of jade, emerald and malachite.

The clarity of the heart chakra is in direct relation to how much heavenly light is shining and descending into the lower earthly chakras. YAM.

Fifth Chakra Balancing

Jing—Neck movement and relaxation. King draws sword. Opening of C7. Because is related to the thyroid, the use of setu bandha sarvangasana or salamba sarvangasana. Theses are the the "mother of all poses" used for spinal opening, clearing of C7, gentle compression on the thyroid, reverse flow of blood circulation, and also opens the Governing Vessel at the Kiln of Dao. Many of the seated Eight Pieces of Brocade exercises. Adho Mukha Vrksasana.

Qi—learning to speak satya or truths. You become what you repeatedly say (and you say the thoughts you loop). Use of blue topaz, lapis and lazuli. Sound reverbs. Mantras. Lymphatic massage. Gargling, brushing, and rinsing with Taoist salt.

Shen—following one's dreams, and use of personal power to manifest in the world. Finding balanced self-expression. Mastering of speech for clear and concise communication so as to not be misunderstood.

Sixth Chakra Balancing

Jing—Adho Mukha Vrksasana and sirsasana. Small circuit movement such as the Golden Qi Ball

Qi—Cherishing the One meditation, the inner light meditation, the inner smile meditation, stones of amethyst and turquoise. Taoist salt protocols for the face openings—washing eyes, netti pot, mouth wash, moist ear swabs. Nadi shodhan pranayama (alternate nostril breathing) to balance the flow of the right and left hemispheres of the brain.

Shen—working to balance right and left brain, or the masculine and feminine aspects of self. Willingness to evaluate self in compassionate ways. Building of intuition and knowledge, proper use of intellect, openness to new ideas.

Seventh Chakra Balancing

Jing—Sirsasana. Small circuit movement.

Qi—1-10 meditation, diamonds and quartz crystals.

Shen—trusting in the compassionate nature of the spirits. Acquiring a positive attitude, values, ethics, and courage. Finding balanced humanitarianism, looking for the larger patterns in life. Finding the polarity to see non-polarity to access the infinite knowledge of wuji. Visualizing one's higher self for a place of spiritual sanctuary and inner peace.

Part 8

Eight Trigrams, Eight Vessels, Eight Limbs of Yoga

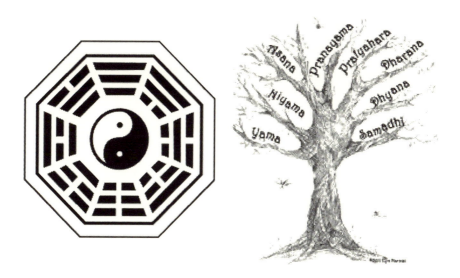

The Eight Trigrams

A person could dedicate his or her whole life to the study of the Eight Trigrams. A basic understanding, however, will give you what you need to benefit from Qi Gong and Zen Yoga training. The Trigrams represent the movement of time, energy, and matter. To understand this is to understand the laws of the universe or the Tao. "He who understands the Tao is sustained by the Tao. He who does not is consumed by the Tao."

Our goal as human beings is to live in harmony with self, others and the universe. The practice of Zen Yoga and Qi Gong is a time-tested method of achieving this goal.

It is best to start at the beginning. The Trigrams begin with nothing. That is known as Wu Ji. This is a state of formlessness or, as Western science would say, the super field. From nothing comes all things. This is the state of Tai Chi or formless energy. For energy to become form you need polarity, also known as the two poles of yin and yang. The two poles yield the four phases. The four phases generate the Eight Trigrams.

The *Zhou Yi* says that Tai Chi was originally misty and turbid, having no shape, no Yi (i.e., intention of change). But there is one qi within. When this qi circulates in the universe, all places are reached. All living things are originated. The "one qi" is also called Pre-Heaven Real Sole Qi. From this qi, the two poles (yin and yang) were generated and heaven and earth began to divide. Since then the yin and yang have been distinguished from each other.

From the yin contracting inward to the yang expanding outward, the trigrams are three lines stacked on top of each other to show the eight arrangement options of yin and yang. Starting with all three lines moving outward, yang energy, then next the top yang line weakens first to yin (like the roof of a house). As the yin drops down, the lower lines adjust accordingly.

Each of the arrangements of three lines, or trigram, has a name for its symbolic meaning, such as Heaven, Earth, Wind, Mountain, Valley, Thunder, Fire, and Water. This allows a word to point to the symbol, not getting lost in the word as a definitive meaning of the symbol, but to offer an idea of what the symbol is expressing.

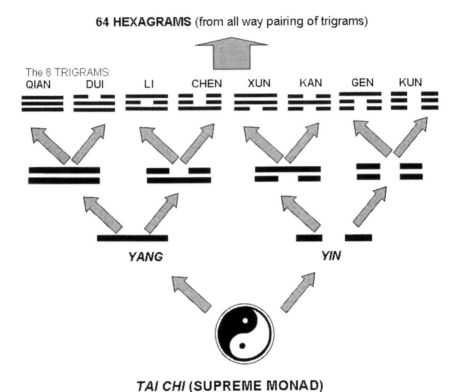

Asanas (postures) may be practiced in assisting the body to feel the expression of the trigram. The postures and trigrams below will aid in becoming familiar and "embodying" the understanding. Multiple trigrams may be placed over the same asana, depending on the focus of the posture series.

Heaven is heaven-like energy, running upward and outward in motion. One yang line stacking on top of another to full lift. One would view the heavens as up and vastly expansive, especially when viewing the night sky when the atmosphere is not catching the reflection of the sun's rays off the surface of the earth. Yang would be light, and daytime is obvious. At night the only natural light comes from the heavens ... stars, planets, moon, comets, etc. Non-universal light would be earth light from fire, reflection of light caught in valleys, and lightning in our atmosphere. These are of the Yang Family with some yin inside the trigram to represent that of earth's atmosphere.

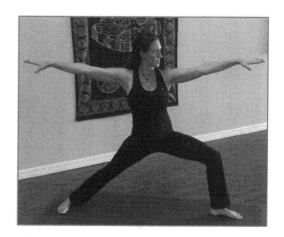

Heaven

Warrior II Pose expands and stretches out from the centerline. The back and shoulders open as the waist opens and feet expand away from the centerline.

Earth is the opposite or polarity of heaven with all three of its lines being yin, and the most yin of the Yin Family. Earth being the most dense and of actual form. There are four trigrams that belong to the Yin Family just as there are four that belong to the Yang Family. Each of the Yin Family trigrams keep the baseline as yin, and the yang family keeps the baseline as yang. How the lines are arranged show how light or heavy the trigram is, and where within the trigram the yin and yang are expressed.

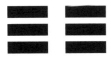

Earth

Press the palms together and contract the chest. Lift the knee and close the centerline. Grab the earth with each toe and root the body.

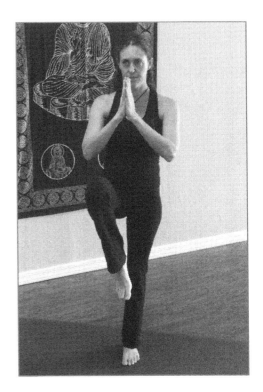

Yang Family

Heaven—see above.

Valley

From the full light of heaven comes the first entry of yin or earth element into the yang mixture. With two yang lines on bottom and one yin line on top, the symbol of Valley contains the light of heaven in its basin. Still highly ethereal—yet the beginning decent of yin though the heaven's yang, bringing it just to the point where it touches the earth. The place of heaven meeting earth is Valley. (Also, referenced as Lake.) This would be equivalent to the heavens opening up as rain falls and filling the valley to become the lake.

Valley

Warrior I Pose. Draw the shoulders up and in. The waist opens as the feet expand away from the centerline.

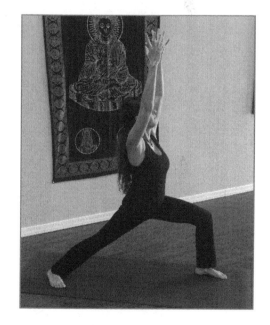

Fire

Showing with the yin in the center line donating the outward glow of light from a consuming of inner yin. This would be the light between heaven and earth. the campfire built from earth reaching upward toward the heaven. With the bottom and top lines as yang, and the center drawn as yin. Still a fair amount of light is being expressed.

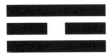

Fire

Upward Facing Dog pose integrates your legs with your entire spine. Lift the chest forward and up. Contract the lower back. The thigh bones are strongly lifting from the floor.

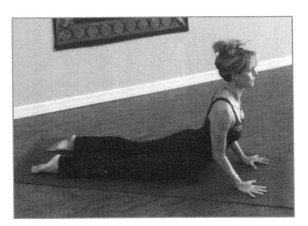

Thunder

The least of the yang family with a yang line still at the base position, but with both above lines stacked heavy with yin. The yang here is showing the movement across the bottom rumbling within the earth.

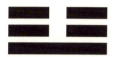

Thunder

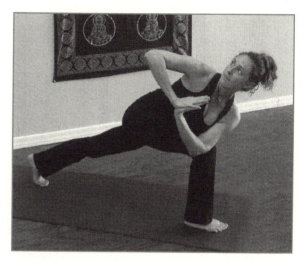

Twisted Crescent Pose. Draw the shoulders down and to the center. Contract the abdomen. Close the hips. Roll the thighs inward to turn the feet into the earth.

Yin Family

Earth—see above.

Water
Yin and shapable on the top and bottom lines, yet a current of movement and strength in the center line. Water symbology here is the hidden danger of water. Like a wave of ocean water that seems gentle and misting on the outer mask, and deep below the wave dark stillness, while the middle of the wave may possess the strength to press things in the direction of its current.

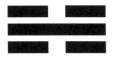

Water

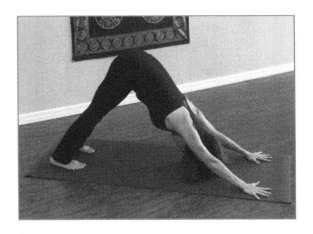

Downward Facing Dog soothes the nervous system as you fully extend your body. The shoulder blades contract and pull toward the pelvis. The sides of the waist elongate. The thigh bones are grounding toward the hamstrings.

Mountain

Seen as solid earth below with the heavens at the top. You look up at a mountain, and down into a valley. Being drawn with the two bottom lines as yin, and the top line as yang, the symbol looks much like a sturdy table.

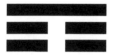

Mountain

Twisted Triangle Pose. Extend the front of the body and open the chest. Contract the abdomen and twist the waist. Roll the thighs inward to turn the feet into the earth.

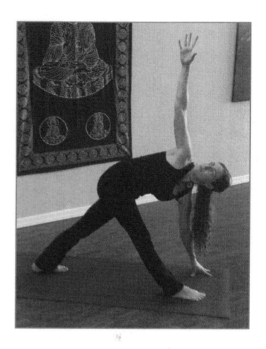

Wind

Being the least yin, yet still holding to the Yin Family value of a contracting line as the base and above both stacked lines are yang to show the movement of wind. Wind moves above the earth's surface. If you look at the different atmospheric currents it will show the pattern of wind moving above the earth up into the top of our bubble.

Wind

Triangle Pose. Open the arms and expand the chest. Lift the knee and open the hips. Grip the earth with each toe and root into the earth.

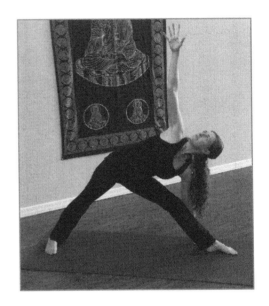

Part 8: Eight Trigrams, Eight Vessels, Eight Limbs of Yoga

What Are the Pre- & Post-Heaven Arrangements?

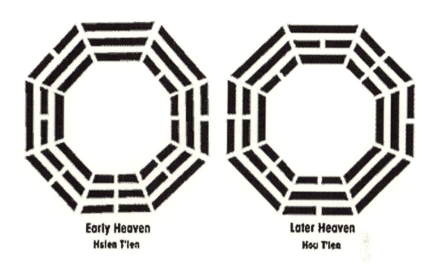

Early Heaven
Hsien T'ien

Later Heaven
Hou T'ien

Pre-Heaven (Early Heaven) Arrangement places the trigrams across from their opposite or polarity trigram to show the balanced state of heaven. Pre=heaven is before form, and without the sin. Sin derived from the greek archer's word for missing the mark. The amount of sin was the measure from the center to where the arrow pierced. The sin is the imperfection of form. This arrangement places each trigram with its opposite: Heaven and Earth, Fire and Water, Valley and Mountain, and Thunder and Wind.

The Post-Heaven (Later Heaven) Arrangement is not balanced. Instead it groups the trigrams in families and shows how the time, energy, and matter changes and moves once in form. It begins with Fire over Water. This is one of the most profound combinations. Flipped it becomes Water over Heaven. One can argue that the trigram on top is dependent on the point of view or perspective from which it is viewed. For this application, it will be discussed as viewed from inside the circle. The order of the trigrams when starting with Fire on top and moving counterclockwise around the circle called the Ba Gua is Wind, Thunder, Mountain, Water, Heaven, Valley, and Earth.

The use of the Eight Trigrams and their arrangement within the Ba Gua are often associated with the chart below when applied to feng shui.

Eight Trigram Attribute Chart

Name	Image	Family Member	Body Part	Illness, Injury	Element	Compass Direction	Star Number
Chien	Heaven	Father (CEO, Owner)	Head Lungs	Head, Pulmonary	Metal	Northwest	6
Kun	Earth	Mother, Matriach	Abdomen, Womb	Digestive, abdominal	Earth	Southwest	2
Chen	Thunder	Eldest Son	Legs, Feet, Throat	Legs, Throat, Hysteria	Wood	East	3
Kan	Deep Abyss	Middle Son, Middle Aged Man	Ears, Kidney	Vertigo, Kidney, Bladder, Blood	Water	North	1
Ken	Mountain	Youth, Youngest son	Hands, Arms, Back	Hand, arm, small bones	Earth	Northeast	8
Sun	Penetrating Wind	Eldest Daughter	Buttocks	Hips, thighs, buttocks	Wood	Southeast	4
Li	Illuminating Fire	Middle Daughter, Middle Aged Woman	Eyes, Heart	Eye disease or injury, Heart problems	Fire	South	9
Tui	Joyous Marsh	Youngest Daughter, Women	Mouth, Chest	Injury illness to mouth or chest	Metal	West	7

Each of the Eight Trigrams relate to the chakras, taking the idea that the Heaven trigram belongs to the seventh chakra and the Earth trigram is the base on which the other six rest upon. Since the seventh chakra is actually above our heads and therefore outside our physical body, there are only six chakras that reside in the body, leaving the eighth trigram of Earth as our true foundation. The idea is that when the soul exits the body (at death), it either ascends into the seventh Heaven chakra or descends into the hell of Earth to repeat an earthly existence to finish outstanding karma. For humans, consciousness may "awaken," as it sleeps in rocks and minerals, dreams in plants, and stirs in creatures. This "awakening" means achieving the ability to reside in the seventh chakra (Heaven), which can happen while in this body or at death. Each person is said to be gifted with at least three glimpses into the seventh chakra—pure "ah-ha" moments. The rest have to be cultivated to achieve samadhi or zen. You may notice that the interior of the body has six chakras. These each correspond to a line in a hexagram (two trigrams stacked on each other). The lines start between the first and second chakras and go upward. This leaves the heart chakra between the lower trigram (Earthly) and the upper trigram (Heavenly)—so humanity divides Heaven and Earth. Contemplate this using the chart below.

CHIEN	☰	111	7	White	SAHASRARA	Above Crown		SUN	ABOVE WHEEL
TUI	☱	110	6	Purple	AJNA	3rd Eye		MOON	Leo/Cancer
LI	☲	101	5	Blue	VISHUDDHA	Throat		MERCURY	Virgo/Gemini
XUN	☴	100	4	Green	ANAHATA	Heart		VENUS	Libra/Taurus
CHEN	☳	011	3	Yellow	MANIPURA	Navel		MARS	Scorpio/Aries
KAN	☵	010	2	Orange	SWADHISTHANA	Sacral		JUPITER	Sagittarius/Pisces
KEN	☶	001	1	Red	MULADHARA	Root		SATURN	Capricorn/Aquarius
KUN	☷	000	0	Black	BRAHMA	Below Feet		EARTH	BELOW WHEEL

What Are the Eight Extraordinary Vessels?

Within Chinese Medicine, "vessels" are the deepest energetic structure within the body, acting as reservoirs or storage containers for qi. These vessels gather extra qi from the Twelve Meridians or primary channels when in excess, or give out qi when there is a deficit. Vessels are also called the Extraordinary Meridians and thus balance and regulate the body's qi flow. These are divided into four pairs. The chong mai and yin wei mai, the du mai and yang qiao mai, the dai mai and yang wei mai, and the ren mai and yin qiao mai. They locate around the body to hold up its energetic structure.

How are they formed?

The vessels develop while in utero, beginning with the joining of the egg and sperm to first create the Thrusting vessel or Tai Ji Pole, then the Governing and Conception vessels, followed by the Belt vessel for the external energy formations.

The secondary formations of vessels are responsible for the internal embryonic tissues and are comprised of the Yin Linking, Yang Linking, Yin Heel and Yang Heel vessels.

The Governing, Conception and Thrusting vessels circulate qi and aid the wei chi field. Conception and Thrusting govern the body's life cycle by moving jing. Each vessel governs an internal connection. The brain is governed by the Governing and Yin and Yang Heel vessels. The uterus by the Thrusting and Conception vessels. Blood vessels by the Thrusting vessel. Gall bladder by the Belt vessel. Marrow by the Thrusting vessel and bones by the Thrusting and Conception vessels.

The specific vessels belonging to the "Eight Extras" family are: 1) Du Mai (Governing Vessel), 2) Ren Mai (Conception Vessel), 3) Chong Mai (Thrusting Vessel), 4) Dai Mai (Belt Vessel), 5) Yang Chiao Mai (Yang Motility Vessel), 6) Yin Chiao Mai (Yin Motility Vessel), 7) Yang Wei Mai (Yang Regulating Vessel), and (8) Yin Wei Mai (Yin Regulating Vessel).

The Governing Vessel (Greater Yang)

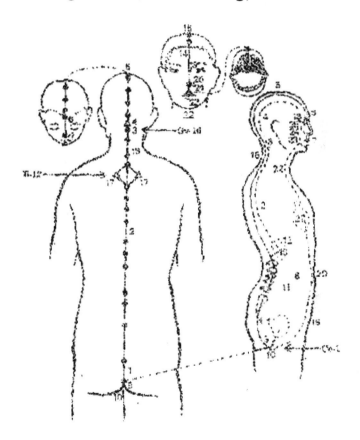

The Governing Vessel includes four courses and is the confluence of all the yang channels over which it is said to "govern." Because it controls all the yang channels, it is called the "Sea of Yang Meridians." This is apparent from the pathway because it flows on the midline of the back, (a yang area and in the center of all yang channels—except the stomach channel which flows in the front). Since the Governing Vessel governs all yang channels, it can be used to increase the yang energy of the body. The Governing Vessel flows from the upper lip over the head down the middle of the back to the perineum (hui yin). How do they manifest disorder? A closed or unraveling Governing Vessel is opened with master point SI3 when showing signs of mania-depression, epilepsy, occipital headache, and stiffness of pain of the spinal column. Opening of the Governing Vessel is also used to dispel febrile diseases and external wind cold or wind heat.

The Conception Vessel (Greater Yin)

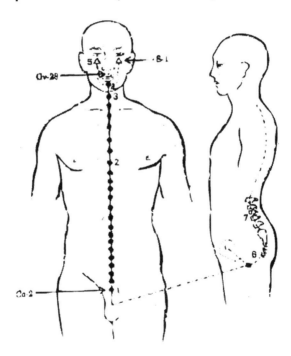

The Conception Vessel has a major role in qi circulation, directing and being responsible for all of the yin channels. This vessel includes two courses that nourish the uterus and whole genital system. The Conception Vessel contains both blood and essence (jing) and flows up to the face and around the mouth. This vessel flows from the perineum (hoi yin) up the middle of the front of the body to the lower lip. Conception Vessel is opened with master point LU7 when unbalanced symptoms of the uterus, reproduction, and urinary arise.

The Thrusting Vessel

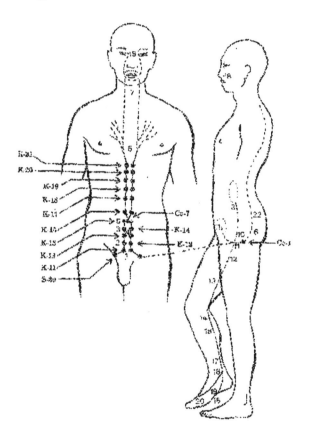

The Thrusting Vessel runs parallel to the kidney meridian of Foot-Shaoyin up to the infra-orbital region. Meeting all the twelve main meridians. It is termed the "Sea of the Twelve Meridians," or the "Sea of Blood." Its function is to reservoir the qi and blood of the twelve main meridians. Thrusting Vessel is opened with the SP4 point to address acute abdominal pain (with cramping), vomiting, and edema (especially of the face).

The Belt Vessel

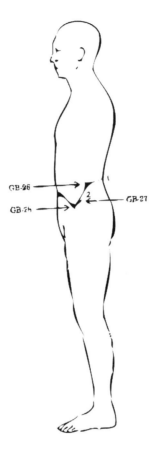

The Belt Vessel originates in the hypochondrium and goes around the waist as a girdle. It performs the function of binding up all the meridians. Being the only horizontal vessel (seen as the equator of the planet earth), the Belt Vessel governs the entire body's qi circulation by encircling and connecting the main channels. Belt Vessel is opened using the master point GB41 to treat breast abscesses, pain, and distention of the breast and menstrual disorders.

The Yang and Yin Heel Vessels

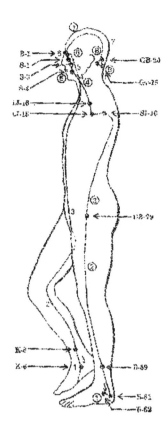

The Yang Heel Vessel starts in the lateral aspect of the heel and merges into the meridian of the Foot-Taiyang to ascend, while the Yin Heel Vessel starts in the medial aspect of the heel and merges into the meridian of the Shaoyin to go upwards. Following their own courses, the two vessels meet each other at the inner canthus. Motion regulation of the lower body is their joint function. Yin and Yang Heel vessels supporting the two lateral sides of the body from the heel up to the eyes. Thus controlling the condition of the muscles in the legs and the muscles that open and close the eyes. Yang Heel Vessel's master point of UB62 treats external and internal wind invasion that shows external wind invasion symptoms such as stiff neck and internal wind invasion including insomnia, lockjaw, opisthotonos, wind stroke, epilepsy, upward staring eyes, deviations of the mouth and eyes or hemiplegia. Yin Heel Vessel is opened with master point KD6 to treat tightness and contraction of the inner aspect of the legs, chronic throat disorders, eyes, and daytime epilepsy.

The Yang and Yin Linking Vessels

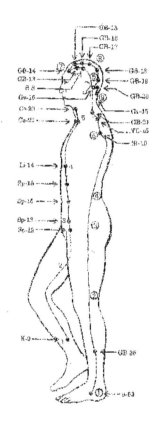

The Yang Linking Vessel is connected with all yang meridians and dominates the exterior of the whole body; the Yin Linking Vessel is connected with all the yin meridians and dominates the interior of the body. The two meridians regulate the flow of qi in the yin and yang meridians, and help maintain coordination and equilibrium between the yin and yang meridians. Yang Linking Vessel uses master point TW5 to treat temporal, frontal, occipital and vertex headaches. Yin Linking Vessel master point PC6 treats pain in the heart and chest, and pain in the lateral costal regions.

Each of the vessels relate to specific indications found within the mind and body. By studying the indications of imbalance and asanas (postures) to rebalance, one may manage many common conditions of life. Below are a few indications and sample asanas for the four vessels that touch all meridians.

Conception Vessel: Opens with Lung 7 and Kidney 6. Relates to responsibility for, or fostering of, the process of birth, whether that be a child, creative idea or endeavor. Therefore, it regulates the uterus, menstruation, menopause, pregnancy, etc. Since the master point is on the Lung channel, it is associated with respiratory syndromes, e.g., childhood asthma. Useful in addressing breathing imbalances.

ASANA: Heart and Lung openers. Cow pose, Cobra, Up Dog.

Governing Vessel: Opens with SI3 and UB62. This meridian pair is effective in treating stiffness in the shoulder, neck, and back, and also regulates the inner canthus of the eye. When this coupling of meridians is utilized in treatment, the entire spine is addressed. It also nourishes the brain, and treats dizziness and tinnitus. On an energetic level, the Du relates to transformational cycles, survival issues, and being grounded in the world. Psycho-spiritually, issues of becoming "upright" and independent, as well as risk-taking, are relevant.

ASANA: Spine lengthening, Down Dog, forward bends, Cat.

Belt Vessel: Opens with GB41 and TW5. The Dai Mai treats the lateral side of the torso, but also can treat problems in the shoulders and lateral side of the neck. The Dai Mai is functionally paired with the Yang Wei Mai, and treated together these channels can work with a lot of classic Shaoyang symptoms like alternating chills and fever and flank pain or fullness. It's short, encircling the body approximately at the waistline. It is structurally paired with the Chong Mai, so is often discussed when considering women's disorders. It can easily be associated with the point called Dai Mai, GB26—a point primarily used for transforming damp heat, particularly when there is a problem of discharge from the lower jiao.

ASANA: Any twisting postures and core work.

Thrusting Vessel: Opens with SP4 and PC6. The Chong Mai is said to link up the twelve regular channels' blood and qi to a greater degree than the other extraordinary channels. The Chong runs through the core of the body and has a great influence on the menstruation of female bodied people, storing the blood as the cycle progresses towards the monthly flow. It is sometimes called the "Sea of Blood."

ASANA: Internal lengthening such as Tadasana or Tree Pose.

Part 8: Eight Trigrams, Eight Vessels, Eight Limbs of Yoga

Below are the Master Points for the four main vessels. Upon knowing the location of each point on the body, meditate by seeing all sixteen points at one time (points are bilateral so there will be two locations per point mentioned).

	Master Point	Coupled Point
Governing/Du Mo	SI3	BL62
Yang Qiao	Bl62	SI3

****

Conception/Ren Mo	LU7	KI6
Yang Qiao	Kl6	LU7

****

Belt/Dai Mo	GB41	TW5
Yang Wei	TW5	GB41

****

Thrusting / Chong Mo	SP4	PC6
Yang Qiao	PC6	SP4

****

What Are the Eight Limbs of Yoga?

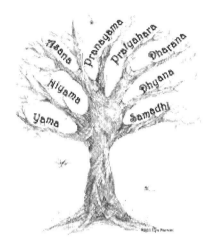

Yama
Niyama
Asana
Pranayama
Pratyahara
Dharana
Dhyana
Samadhi

"The right means are just as important as the end in view." Patanjali enumerates these means as the eight limbs or stages of yoga for the quest of the soul.

From *Light on Yoga* and *Hatha Yoga Pradipika*—B.K.S. Iyengar.

1) Yama are universal moral commandments, also referred to as "restraints." Used to mentally set the mind for a yoga practice. They are divided into five parts known as:

Ahimsa: Non-violence, loving yourself and others, gentleness, justice, no pride nor fear.

Satya: Truthfulness, being true to your nature. Seeking and speaking truth.

Asteya: Non-stealing, not keeping for yourself when others lack. Recognizing the beauty in simplicity.

Bramacharya: Moderation in all things, in body, mind and speech.

Aparigraha: Non-possessiveness, not hoarding, feeling no loss. ("I have all that I need")

2) Niyama: self-purification by discipline, the development of yogic virtues seen in five parts:

Saucha: Inner as well as outward cleanliness, positive thoughts and actions. Benevolence.

Santosa: Contentment with self. Gratitude, feeling no lack. Tranquility.

Tapas: Fiery cleansing. Recognizing each experience as an opportunity to let go. Equanimity.

Savadhyaya: Study of the self in its highest form. Seeking knowledge.

Isvara Pranidhana: Devotion to the divine. Recognizing the divine in all. Surrender to god.

3) Asana, or postures, are physically done in a yoga practice. Asana keep the body healthy and strong and in harmony with nature. Ultimately the yogini becomes free of physical consciousness. The body is the temple of god, and the yogi is god (or at least an aspect of the divine). Through asana practice, the body becomes a fit vehicle for the soul. Through asana the practitioner opens the body and breaks through blocks (granthis) as a means of breaking through psychological blocks and conditioned thoughts and behavior (samsara). The three major blocks (granthis) are attachment to possessions, attachment to people, and thinking of oneself as special or unique—having special abilities. Asana develops a strong and elastic body, soothes the nerves, and enables the practitioner to assume focus and stability of the mind.

These three (Yama, Niyama, & Asana) are the first stages in the outward quests (Brahiranga Sadhana).

The next two stages of yoga (or limbs) teach the aspiring yogi to regulate the breath and their mind. This helps to free the senses from the plethora of objects of desire and are inner quests (Antaranga Sadhana).

4) Pranayama, or breath observation, expansion

Prana means breath, respiration, life, vitality, wind, energy, and strength. It also implies the soul vs. the body. The word is generally plural —"ayama" of vital breaths. Meaning to lengthen, expand, stretch, or restrain. Pranayama suggests extending and controlling the breath. Control of all functions of breathing, including: 1) inhalation or inspiration, or to fill up (puraka); 2) exhalation or expiration of emptying the lungs (rechaka); 3) retention or holding the breath, a state of no inhalation or exhalation (kumbhaka).

Pranayama is the science of breath. Exampled by viewing a pitcher, water pot, jar, or chalice. This container may be full of water, or emptied and filled with air. Prana is meant to be brought under control in a slow progression to match one's capacity and physical ability. Life is not measured in days, but instead in breaths. Focusing on observing the breath's expansion and contraction helps free the conditioned mind from relentless scanning and analysis (its conditioned thinking).

In pranayama the spine and spinal muscles are the sources of action. The lungs are the receiving instruments.

Pranayama is used for clearing the body of old mucus, bile, and wind (these blockages prevent effective pranayama).

By focusing on the breath, the psychological disturbances that manifest during meditation—impurity, distraction, ignorance, dullness, delusion, and scattered thinking—may be harnessed and stilled.

Hasta or Hand Mudras (gesture/seal) in pranayama are used to both hold the mind to a focused inward position as well as to emphasize and improve effects of breath control. Prana increased to specific areas as desired by controlling the position of the hands, thus revealing strain in the muscles responsible for each breath movement with visualization to the desired region, as well as steadying the mind. Mudras are done with different positioning of the hands, and with emphasis on the thumb (lung meridian). Qi radiates from the fingertips, which have Jing (Well) points found in the Jing well therapy protocol in part 12. Through the use of hand mudras, the qi then moves through these circuits, aiding in calming, centeredness, devotion, and so on. Making the circuits complete and bringing flexibility to the wrists, hands, and fingers connects the circuits on a jing, qi, and shen level.

5) Pratyahara (withdrawal of the senses)

Wood—Sight
Fire—Taste
Earth—Touch
Metal—Smell
Water—Sound
Qi Fire—Intuition

When we lose reason to our senses it causes qi to travel outward. The cutting off of the senses is to keep the qi within. *"To sever the use of one sense is ten thousand times better than employing a teacher."*

By closing the eyes our sight is to be turned to our inner light and images, which can be soothing or disruptive. When the senses are open to the outside world, one is compelled or repelled by that which is in the field of influence. Each charge running toward or from an external influence draws on one's qi reserves. We are constantly pulled by our sense desires—the tastes we love and seek, the smells that remind us of past memories, the longing for connecting touch, sounds that move us. When there is rhythmic control over the breath, we no longer run after these external objects of desire. Turning inward frees us from the power of the senses. In this stage the seeker (sadhaka) goes inward, searching through self-examination. To overcome the deadly and attractive spell of sensual objects, we need the insulation of devotion and adoration (bahkti) by recalling our mind as the creator that created all of the objects of our desires. While practicing withdrawing from the senses, you become free of ego and attachment as you sees yourself as the divine self (Atman). Turning inward, you notice the conditioning of self, removing from reaction to stimuli and instead observing your conditioned responses and selective attention. "What am I conditioned to notice?" By mastering pratyahara, one transcends the dualities of pleasure and pain, becoming fearless, generous, self-controlled, nonviolent, truthful, tranquil, charitable, gentle, modest, steady, illuminated, and free from pride.

6) Dharana (controlling one's senses)

Once the physical self is tempered by asana, the mind refined from the fiery pranayama, and the senses are under control through the practice of pratyahara, the seeker (sadhaka) reaches the sixth stage called Dharana. In this stage there is pinpoint focus and concentration when being engrossed in a task. Here the mind must be stilled in order to reach this state of complete absorption. To the extent that one transcends the dualistic relationship of the subject (me) observing the object (other), and becomes one with what is contemplated or the "I am" (Yahweh). This is the basis of Tantra, the dissolve of measurement, judgement, and comparison in contemplation of the breath, the universal energies, a flower's color or scent, a sound, and so forth. The training of the "Monkey Mind."

7) Dhyana (meditation)

This stage of yoga brings the sadhaka to a yogi's clear mind. The mind like water shapes to its container. When contemplating an object the mind becomes the shape of that object. Holding the view of divinity, which it worships, ultimately through long-continued devotions, the mind is then transformed into the likeness of divinity. Uninterrupted flow of light or mind meditation on the divine illuminates the yogi's mind to dhyana. Progress on the path of yoga shows as good health, sense of physical lightness, steadiness, clearness of features and eyes, beautiful voice, sweet odor of the body, and freedom from craving, then one has a balanced, serene, and tranquil mind.

8) Samadhi (meditative absorption)

The sadhaka's quest peaks in meditation at the passing into samadhi, where the body and senses are at rest as if sleeping, faculties of mind and reason are alert as if awake, and one is beyond consciousness. The person in a state of samadhi is fully conscious and alert. The soul within the heart is smaller than the smallest seed, yet greater than the sky, containing all works, all desires. Into this the sadhaka enters. Then there remains no sense of "I" or "mine" as the working of the body. The mind and the intellect have stopped as if one is in deep sleep. The sadhaka has attained true union (yoga); there is only experience of consciousness, truth, and unutterable joy. There is a peace that passes all understanding. There are no thoughts. The result of having trained the "Monkey Mind" to sit still enables one to sit with the "Universal Mind."

Part 9

Nine Gates & Three Hearts

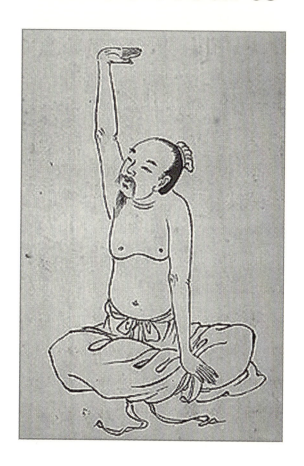

Zen Wellness
Three Hearts & Nine Gates Medical Qi Gong

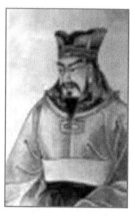

The Zen Wellness Three Hearts & Nine Gates Medical Qi Gong training protocol finds its roots in the Eight Pieces of Brocade set developed by General Yu Fei. He mandated that all his officials, officers, and troops start every day with a complete Qi Gong protocol. He found his people to be much healthier mentally and physically. This allowed them to live longer, be more productive, and have healthier lives, thus better serving the country.

These eight exercises are used to stimulate the central nervous system, lower blood pressure, relieve stress and gently tone muscles without strain. They also enhance digestion, elimination of wastes, and the circulation of blood.

Making beneficial exercises interesting and enjoyable has always been a challenge to creative people. Hua T'o (110–207 CE) was one of the famous physicians of the Han Dynasty. In *The History of the Later Han,* Hua T'o wrote:

The body must have exercise, but it should never be done to the point of exhaustion. By moving about briskly, digestion is improved, the blood vessels are opened, and illnesses are prevented. It is like a used doorstep which never rots.

What Are the Nine Gates?

The Nine Gates are the major joints of the body. The Gates are looked at in sets of three. The sets can be looked at like a tree with the roots being ankles, knees, hips. The trunk being the lumbar, thoracic, and cervical vertebra, and the wrists, elbows, and shoulders being the branches of a tree. All three sections must be strong, flexible, and lubricated to be healthy. You can break down the smaller joints in the hands and feet in sets of three as well.

One of the objectives of Zen Yoga is to strengthen the tendons that support the joints. By holding yoga positions, you trigger the muscles around the joints. This increases the prana flow around and through the joints.

Many joint problems that occur outside of accidental injury are the product of poor alignment and weak connective tissue. It is common for people to rely on the strength of the ligaments to hold the body in place. As time passes, you slowly strain the ligaments, resulting in many of the joint problems people suffer with today.

The Three Hearts

When referring to the Three Hearts, the first heart that comes to mind is the heart in your chest. By moving the spine and arms in coordination with yogic breathing, the first heart is balanced. To balance the heart is to relieve it of the up-and-down heart rate caused by chest breathing. Chest breathing is easily affected by our emotions. By using the yogic breathing method, we better oxygenate the blood and cause the heart to be more effective and efficient in supplying the body with oxygen.

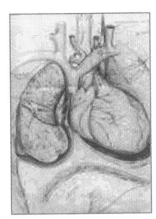

Part 9: Nine Gates & Three Hearts

Lower abdominal breathing is considered the second heart. As the abdomen expands and contracts the organs below the diaphragm are stimulated. This movement has a profound impact on the circulation of fluid and prana supporting digestion and elimination.

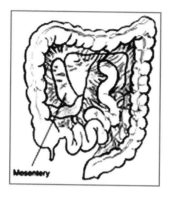

The third heart is the gastrocnemius or calf muscle. By flexing the calf, the blood in the lower body is re-circulated up to the heart. Adding circulation in this manner reduces pressure in the vascular valves reducing risk of varicose veins and edema in the lower body.

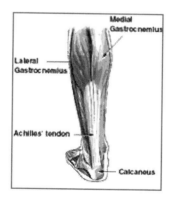

The Three Hearts and Nine Gates are addressed in the Asanas in the following section. Through the movements of the postures, all nine gates are stabilized and the three hearts supported through breath and movement.

Seated Eight Brocades

Primarily focuses on exercising the upper limbs, benefits the six organs, and relates to the six meridians in the arms. Seated Eight Brocades is a great way to wake up and put yourself to bed, or for people who are bedridden or cannot easily stand. (No torso twisting when pregnant.)

Form 1: Holding Mt. Kunlun w/Both Hands

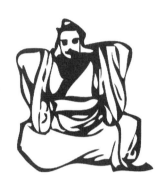

Loosen your belt and clothing. Sit upright on a mat or towel with legs bent, the right calf over the left with both soles facing obliquely upward. Relax your whole body and concentrate your mind, looking straight ahead. Tap your teeth together lightly 36 times, with the tip of the tongue touching the hard palate, and pause briefly. When your mouth becomes filled with saliva, swallow it in three gulps with a gulping sound. Then cover your ears with your palms, fingers spread out like a fan. Place forefingers on middle fingers and tap on the back of the head 24 times. Take a deep breath, inhaling and exhaling slowly and evenly. (Fig. 1).

Form 2: Shaking the Heavenly Pillar

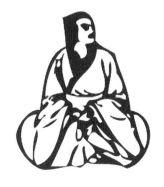

Sit upright with legs bent, right calf over the left, with soles facing obliquely upward. Place right palm on left above navel, with fingers slightly bent. Turn your head to the left, eyes looking backward as far as possible, for one or two seconds (Fig. 2). Then turn your head to the right reversing the positions of the palms. Repeat 24 times. Keep torso erect while turning your head, with chin slightly tucked to align the cervical vertebrae properly.

Form 3: Raising Arms

Sit upright with palms resting on bent knees, right calf over the left, both soles facing obliquely upward, and eyes straight ahead. Make relaxed fists and raise them overhead as if you were hanging from a horizontal bar (Fig. 3). Move your tongue around the inside of your mouth 36 times to produces saliva and swallow this in three audible gulps. Close your eyes and imagine that your heart center (different than the heart organ!) is being warmed by a torch with the flames spreading gradually throughout the whole body. Return palms to knees.

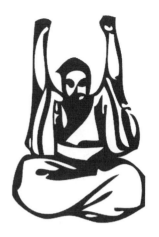

Form 4: Rubbing Lower Back

Strip to waist and sit upright with legs bent, right calf over the left and soles facing obliquely upward. Rub palms together until they are warm and place them on your sides with thumbs pointing forward and fingers pointing obliquely downward (Fig. 4). Rub hands up and down at lease 36 times against both sides of spinal cord. Put on your garment and place left palms below navel, right palms on back of left hand. Breathe gently and imagine a flame in your lower heart center spreading down to the region below the navel. You feel warm all over.

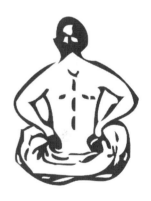

Form 5: Twisting the Torso to the One Side

Sit as in Form 4 with right hand on hip and left palm on abdomen above navel, eyes looking straight ahead. Turn left shoulder forward and right shoulder backward, and then return to original position. Repeat 36 times, turning head together with shoulders.

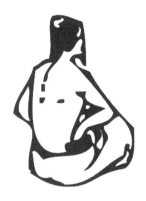

Form 6: Twisting the Torso to Both Sides

Sit as in Form 4. Turn left shoulder forward and right shoulder backward, and then reverse this motion. Repeat 36 times, gradually increasing degree of rotation (Fig. 6). Place left palm on lower abdomen, and rest the right palm on back of the left hand. Close your eyes gently and imagine a flame spreading from the lower abdomen up to the waist and then continuing up between the shoulder blades to the top of the head. Stretch legs forward, toes pointing up and muscles relaxed. Close your mouth lightly and take three deep breaths through your nose.

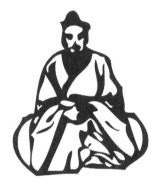

Form 7 Propping Up the Sky with Fingers Interlocked

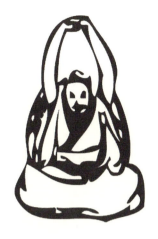

Sit upright with legs bent, right calf over the left, both soles facing obliquely upward. With palms facing upwards, lock fingers together, pressing the little fingers against abdomen. Look straight ahead. Raise palms to chest level and then above head while gradually twisting wrists until palms face upward (Fig. 7). Then return palms to abdomen. Repeat nine times, inhaling when raising palms and exhaling when lowering them. Sit upright with legs stretched forward, feet shoulder-width apart. Place palms on floor at your sides with thumbs touching the body and fingers pointing forward. Look straight ahead.

Form 8: Pulling Toes with Both Hands

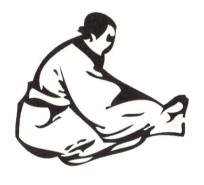

Bend forward and grasp the ball and toes of one foot with both hands, pulling back the top of the foot as you thrust the heel forward. Repeat with other foot. Eyes should follow the moving foot. Repeat 12 times, taking a deep breath each time (Fig. 8). Sit quietly for a few moments with eyes and mouth gently closed. Move you tongue around inside your mouth to produce saliva and swallow it quickly. Repeat six times. Then shrug your shoulders and twist your waist. Finally, relax your whole body.

Part 10

Asanas (Postures)

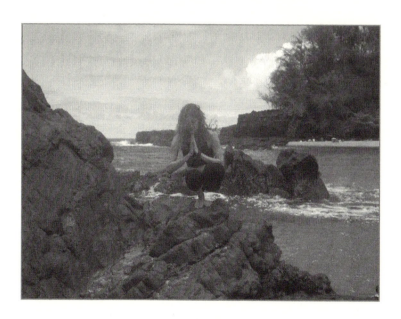

The mixing of Kan and Li method will be used throughout the Zen Yoga practice, with special emphasis when performing the Up Dog and Down Dog positions. The following is a detailed explanation of the breathing method as it applies to this and all movements in the Zen Yoga system.

Zen Yoga
Sixteen Posture System and Eight Trigrams

1. Wuji—Standing Stillness
2. Kan—Water
3. Li—Fire
4. Warrior 1—Valley
5. Warrior 2—Heaven
6. Mix Kan and Li
7. Triangle—Heaven
8. Twisted Triangle—Mountain
9. Mix Kan and Li
10. Crane—Earth
11. Tree—Wind
12. Mix Kan and Li
13. Open Crescent [6th Chi—Electricity]
14. Twisted Crescent—Thunder
15. Mix Kan and Li
16. Sitting Nei Gong Meditation—Mixing Kan and Li

Zen Yoga Flow

Presence / Centering
Pranayama & Rag Doll

Awakening
Sun Salutation A x 3
Sun Salutation B x 3

Vitality
Warrior Twisting Series:
Crescent Lunge
Revolving Crescent Lunge
Extended Side Angle (Arms Extended)
Standing Prayer Twist
Grab Big Toes, Stretch Down, Palm the Earth
Repeat opposite side

Equanimity:
Balancing
Tree
Crane to Warrior III
Standing Padagustasana
Repeat other side

Grounding:
Triangle series
Warrior I
Warrior II
Triangle
Ardha Chandrasana
Twisted Triangle
Vinyasa
Repeat other side

Igniting:
Back Bending Series:
Locust/Bow
Camel
Bridge/Wheel

Stability:
Ab Series:
Plank/Side Plank
Rejuvenation:
Inversion Series:
Shoulder Stand w/vairations
Release:
Forward Bending Series:
Seated forward bend
Presence/Surrender:
Savasana

108 Zen Yoga Flow
Section One

1. Tadasana 131
2. Uttanasana 132
3. Four Fingers Press the Earth 134
4. Eka Pada Parsva Uttanasana 135
5. Ardha Uttanasana 136
6. R Anjaneyasana 138
7. R Banarasana (Low Straight Lunge) 139
8. R Utthan Pristhasana (Lizzard) 141
9. Phalakasana 142
10. Chaturanaga Dandasana 143
11. Bhujangasana (Cobra) 144
12. Balasana 145
13. Marjaryasana (Cat)/Bitilasana (Cow) 146
14. Adho Mukha Svanasana/Cat Stretch 148
15. R Vasisthasana to Camatkarasana 149
16. R Tri Pada Adho Mukha Svanasana 150
17. L Vasisthasana to Camatkarasana 151
18. L Tri Pada Adho Mukha Svanasana 151
19. L Anjaneyasana 151
20. L Banarasana 151
21. L Utthan Pristhasana (Lizzard) 151
22. R Urdhva Prasarita Ekapadasana 152
23. L Urdhva Prasartia Ekapadasana 152
24. Malasana 153
25. Bakasana 154
26. Utkatasana 155
27. Samastitihi 156

Section Two

28. R Alanasana (Crescent Lunge) 158
29. R Virabhadrasana I 159
30. R Baddha Virabhadrasana 160
31. Urdhva Mukha Svanasana 161
32. L Alanasana (Crescent Lunge) 161
33. L Virabhadrasana I 162
34. L Baddha Virabhadrasana 162
35. R Utthita Parsvakonasana 162
36. R Virabhadrasana II 163
37. R Viparita Virabhadrasana I—Reverse Warrior 164
38. R Trikonasana 165
39. R Ardha Chandrasana 167
40. R Ardha Chandra Chapasana 168
41. Throw a Ball 169
42. Horse Stance 170
43. Hold the Moon on a Golden Platter 171
44. L Utthita Parsvakonasana 172
45. L Virabhadrasana II 172
46. L Viparita Virabhadrasana—Reverse Warrior 172
47. L Trikonasana 172
48. L Ardha Chandrasana 172
49. L Ardha Chandra Chapasana 172
50. R Parivrtta Utkatasana 173
51. R Parivrtta Anjaneyasana 174
52. Prasarita Padottanasana 175
53. R Parivrtta Prasarita Padottanasana 176
54. L Parivrtta Prasarita Padottanasana 177
55. L Parivrtta Utkastasana 177

56.	L Parivrtta Anjaneyasana	177
57.	Urdhva Hastasana/Double Palms	178
58.	R Standing Crane	179
59.	R Crane Points to 7 Stars	180
60.	R Hasta Padangusthasana	181
61.	R Vrksasana	182
62.	R Virabhadrasana III	183
63.	R Natarajasana	184
64.	R Garudasana	185
65.	L Standing Crane	185
66.	L Crane Points to 7 Star	186
67.	L Hasta Padangusthasana	186
68.	L Vrksasana	186
69.	L Virabhadrasana III	186
70.	L Natarajasana	186
71.	L Garudasana	186

Section Three

72. Moving 8 Vessels: 7 Stars Press Earth 187
73. Divide Heaven and Earth 188
74. Stand in Ba Pull Bow Shoot Arrow 189
75. Twisted Stance to Push Two Poles 190
76. Crescent Moon 191
77. Ride the Tiger 192
78. Natural Palm Points to 7 Stars 193
79. Gather the Sun to Press the Earth 194
80. Taoist Horse Stance 195
81. R Eka Pada Rajakapotasana Rising Up 196
82. R Eka Pada Rajakapotasana w/Fold 198
83. L Eka Pada Rajakapotasana Rising Up 198
84. L Eka Pada Rajakapotasana w/Fold 198
85. Ustrasana 198
86. Virasana 200
87. Setu Bandha Sarvangasana 201
88. Salamba Sarvangasana 203
89. R Sucirandhrasana 205
90. R Agnistambhasana 206
91. R Gomukhasana 207
92. L Sucirandhrasana 208
93. L Agnistambhasana 208
94. L Gomukhasana 208
95. Navasana 208
96. Dandasana 209
97. Pashimotasana 210
98. R Marichyasana 211
99. L Marichyasana 212

Part 10: Asanas

100. R Janu Sirsasana Fold 212
101. R Parivrtta Janu Sirsasana 213
102. L Janu Sirsasana Fold 214
103. L Parivrtta Janu Sirsasana 214
104. Upavistha Konasana 215
105. Baddha Konasana 216
106. Seated Hold a Qi Ball Breathing/Heal Sounds 217
107. Siddhasana w/Infinity Mudra 218
108. Savasana 219

Destiny & Fate

It is said one's destiny is the highest expression outcome for one's life. Fate is the fatal behavior that stands in destiny's way. Our destiny is to achieve a state of zen (non-attachment, non-judgment, non-resistance) in all that we do from birth to death. Fatal behavior distracts the individual's mind, often from emotional discomfort, creating "bumps" in the road. However, not all bumps are fate—some are challenges asking us to rise to the occasion with the highest integrity and holding to core beliefs of correct action. Often that which is correct is harder than the incorrect.

When viewing life and situations, consider the 108 perspectives of a Master. Expanding from a myopic or singular view of mind, to an ability to "walk in someone else's shoes." Meaning, can you see a situation from more than one viewpoint? As you hike a mountain, you only see one side. Upon reaching the top you see all "108" sides.

A true master is one who has mastered a subject or aspect of self. Some lineages point to a master as one who is unquestionably followed as a supreme leader. Seeking a master is seeking an example of someone on whom you would like to model your own behaviors and abilities. Masters are to be venerated and thanked for their success in showing us that mastery is possible to the most basic of individuals with persistence and devotion to the path of mastery.

Mastering of a subject or aspect includes the ability to see the middle from at least 108 different views. Adequate explanation of these 108 views is what creates a master teacher. Master teachers are in all walks of life and all subjects. Within the wisdom teaching lineage, a true master would make other teachers. One hundred eight teachers graduating under a master shows the master's ability to explain the information or the middle view 108 different ways, as each individual requires a different explanation. Growing from a master to a grandmaster would mean the master's 108 students all become masters in their own right. This exemplifies a well-rounded view of a master.

Part 10: Asanas

To the right, you will see a caduceus. The image is of two snakes intertwining along a central pole or energy. One is not leading the other. Each has its own head. The common mind it follows is the Tao. The Tao may be interpreted as the Wi-Fi broadcast that steers the collective to move as one. Think the "silent voice" that makes all the animals hibernate simultaneously. One animal does not lead the others. They move as one. Remember, as you move through life's path, you might not follow one person per say, you follow the higher power—the collective mind signal of the Tao. By adhering to and practicing the Eight Limbs of Yoga, one may be able to tune into this broadcast of the Tao and move in harmony with the tide.

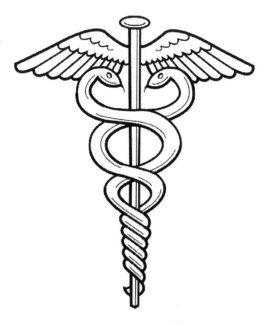

"Only one head on a snake"

Building the Physical Vessel to Hold the Spirit

It is said that the frequency level of the three (jing, qi, shen) will only be as high as the lowest one. So if the mind is strong, the qi is strong, but the body weak; the mind and qi will be weighed down to the frequency of the body. To rise to one's highest potential, all three must be lifted simultaneously. Work on the weakest to achieve the highest.

<u>The posture alignments that follow are meant to be practiced in conjunction with professional instruction. If there is any doubt to your ability to find the alignments, do not practice the postures unless you have a qualified professional to assist. Benefits, cautions, and contraindications will be taught in Zen Yoga Live.</u>

Zen Yoga 108

Section One

1. Tadasana

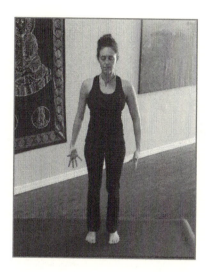

1. While inhaling, lift the crown of the head and lightly tuck the chin to lift the lower occipital ridge, then exhale and descend the tailbone down between the rooting legs and feet.
2. Lengthen the torso by extending the waist and releasing the chest open while keeping the pelvic floor level and heavy.
3. Inhale the shoulders broadened away from the neck by exhaling and drawing the bottom inner tips of the shoulder blades together and in towards the heart.
4. Lift the navel towards the spine and expand the kidneys.

5. Keeping legs weighted and engaged, inhale as you hug and wrap all of the muscles on the legs towards the bones of the legs, then exhale and extend the bones of the legs into the earth as though they are a rooting tree while keeping the tailbone rooted.
6. The legs are straight yet knees are not locked. The thigh bones are turning inward as if corkscrewing the femur into the back of the hip socket. With each inhalation lengthen the torso. With each exhalation bow the torso over the legs.

2. Uttanasana

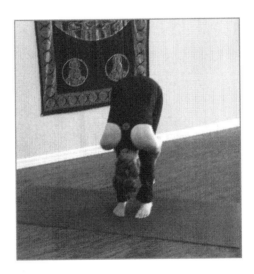

1. Exhale folding at the hips (not the waist) with the hips reaching back gently and allowing the fingers to rest on the floor, block, or holding each elbow with the hands.
2. Inhale and lengthen the waist and torso. Exhale folding more fully into the posture while keeping the neck long and chin slightly tucked.

3. Inhale the shoulders broadened away from the neck by exhaling and drawing the bottom inner tips of the shoulder blades together and in towards the heart.
4. Inhale to lift the navel towards the spine and exhale to expand the kidneys.
5. Keeping legs weighted and engaged, inhale as you hug and wrap all of the muscles on the legs towards the bones of the legs, then exhale and extend the bones of the legs into the earth as though they are a rooting tree while keeping the tailbone rooted.
6. The legs are straight yet knees are not locked. The thigh bones are turning inward as if corkscrewing the femur into the back of the hip socket. With each inhalation lengthen the torso. With each exhalation bow the torso over the legs.
7. Return to standing by bending the knees, placing hands on hips, and inhaling the spine to a vertical position. Exhale to stand by straightening the legs. Stand in tadasana.

3. Four Fingers Press the Earth

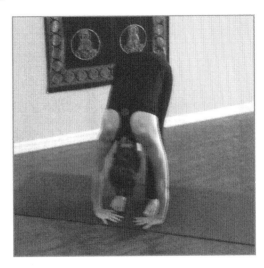

1. Exhale from tadasana, folding at the hips (not the waist) with hips reaching back gently and allow fingers to rest on floor (or block).
2. Inhale and lengthen waist and torso. Exhale folding more fully into the posture while keeping the neck long and chin slightly tucked.
3. With palms flat on floor (or block), transfer weight into the hands while keeping the shoulders broadened away from the neck by drawing the bottom inner tips of the shoulder blades in towards the heart.
4. While moving the weight downward from the heart to the hands and keeping the spine long, maintain the extension of the legs from the lifted core, rooting the tailbone down through the heels.
5. Use the inhales to lengthen and the exhales to fold and press for 1–9 minutes.

6. Come out of the posture on the inhale by bending the knees, sinking the hips to a squat, bringing the spine vertical and exhaling to stand by straightening the legs.
7. Return to tadasana for a few breaths.

4. Eka Pada Parsva Uttanasana

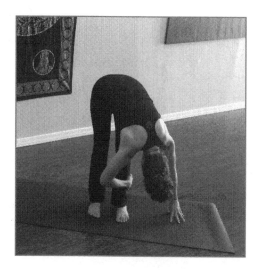

1. Stand with feet parallel and outer hip distance apart. Exhale folding at hips (not waist), gently pulling hips back and setting most of the weight in the heels, rooting through the tailbone while extending the torso.
2. Exhale broadening from navel center towards each side while bowing over thighs, letting the hand reach towards the floor or a block, keeping hips level.
3. Inhale lengthening the spine and waist while rising to fingertips. Draw the navel and torso over the right leg keeping the waist extended. Left hand holds outside of right ankle, right elbow bends while hand touches to the

floor about eight to ten inches outside right foot. Keep the hips level as you exhale.
4. Inhale lengthening spine and waist, once again keeping hips level and chest extended. Exhale into posture.
5. Inhale to come out of twist then exhale while resting the center. Repeat on other side.
6. Come out of the posture on the inhale by bending the knees, sinking the hips to a squat, bringing the spine vertical and exhaling to stand by straightening the legs.
7. Return to tadasana for a few breaths. Repeat on other side.

5. Ardha Uttanasana

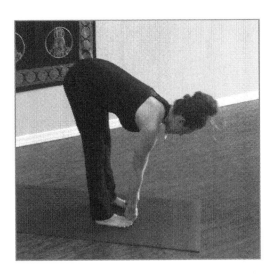

1. Stand with feet parallel and outer hip distance apart. Exhale folding at hips (not waist), gently pulling hips back and setting most of the weight in the heels and rooting through the tailbone while extending the torso and resting the fingertips on the ground.

2. Inhale to extend the waist through the chest to lengthen the lumbar spine and neck, keeping the shoulders broadened away from the neck and exhale pulling the inner scapula towards the heart. Draw the eyes of the elbows in and forward towards your face while holding the big toes.
3. Inhale lifting the torso parallel to the ground and perpendicular to legs while allowing the front chest to broaden and open, then exhale tucking the chin slightly and inhale again to lengthen the vertebrae from lumbar through the neck.
4. Staying in the pose, broaden from the navel center to each side, while keeping the femur bones pulling apart and rotating into the back outer pelvis. Maintain the four pads of the feet firmly on the ground while lifting from the arches up the inner leg to the groin while protecting the kidneys and a slight rolling under of the tailbone.
5. Come out of the posture on the inhale by bending the knees, sinking the hips to a squat, bringing the spine vertical and exhaling to stand by straightening the legs.
6. Return to tadasana for a few breaths.

6. R Anjaneyasana

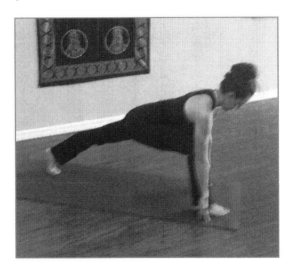

1. From uttanasana, inhale and deeply bend the knees and transfer weight to right leg. Then keeping the hips level, exhale extending the left leg straight back towards rear of mat. Keeping the knee unlocked and pointing the foot at the mat, set it down on the ball of the foot with the heel up and toes on the mat. (IF needed, place the left knee on the mat or blanket instead).
2. While keeping the hips level, inhale stability into the posture by drawing each direction outward from the naval center and exhaling a descending tailbone.
3. Fingertips remain on the ground with one on each side of the forward foot, and without weight in fingers. Use the inhalation to lengthen the torso and side bodies, and the exhalation to soften into the asana. Maintain broadened shoulders and vertebrae reaching from lumbar through occipital ridge while remembering to protect the kidneys.

4. The forward leg holds at a 90-degree angle with knee over ankle and not in front, while back leg is straight and sturdy. Inhale while engaging the muscles onto the legs, and exhale extending into the earth through the feet.
5. Mindfully separate the femur bones from the pelvic floor towards the outer hip while keeping the back leg facing down.
6. To come out of posture, inhale weight into front leg, and exhale sliding the back leg forward next to the front leg.
7. Stand out of the posture on the inhale by bending the knees, sinking the hips to a squat, bringing the spine vertical and exhaling to stand by straightening the legs.
8. Return to tadasana. Then repeat on other side

7. R Banarasana (Low Straight Lunge)

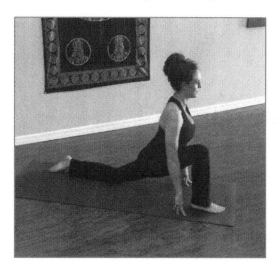

1. From table pose, bring right foot forward towards right hand, placing the lightly expanded foot evenly on floor while keeping the right knee over the right ankle.

1. Relax the left knee and top of the toes onto the floor. Level the pelvis while keeping the hips facing forward.
2. Lengthen the torso up through the heart while keeping the shoulders rolled back and relaxed.
3. Sink into the hips slowly, making sure not to overextend yourself. Find the edge of comfort and rest there for several deep breaths.
4. With a gently tucked chin, feel the earthy heaviness in the hips while lifting vertically up through the body and crown of the head
5. Use blocks under the hands to lessen the intensity of the posture.
6. If a greater stretch is desired, inch the left leg back until you reach the edge of comfort. Never bring the right knee forward past the ankle.
7. Upon completion, return to table pose resting to observe the difference in the quality of right and left hips.
8. Repeat on other side.

8. R Utthan Pristhasana (Lizzard)

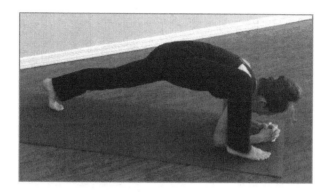

1. From lunge pose with right leg in front, place both hands inside right foot.
2. Keeping the left leg engaged and inner thigh lifting, slowly and cautiously bring the elbows to blocks or the ground.
3. Maintain a lifted buoyant core and engaged tailbone.
4. From the core, extend through the left vertical heel and forward through the heart space.
5. The left leg stays lifted unless a need to modify brings the left knee to the floor.
6. Remain in the posture for multiple breaths.
7. To come out of posture, return to lunge then table. Rest.
8. Repeat on other side.

9. Phalakasana

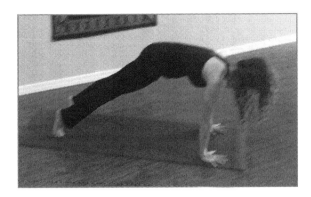

1. From table pose, widely spread your palms as if to suction the hand to the floor. Space your fingers while rooting from the heart through the palm center and keeping your pointer finger's largest knuckle connected firmly.
2. Breathing into the core, visualize the kidney region inflating while keeping the shoulders engaged and heart softened towards the earth.
3. Keeping the shoulders over the wrist, begin to inch the knees back maintaining the core and kidney alignment.
4. On the inhale lift the knees from the floor and straighten the legs while having the bottom of the toes down, and heels directly up.
5. Lighten the posture by lifting in the core and extending forward through the crown of the head, and back through the heels. Press the thigh bones back into the hip sockets and up towards the sky.
6. Breathe for several rounds, then on an exhale release the knees back to the earth and return to table.

10. Chaturanga Dandasana—Four-Limbed Staff Pose

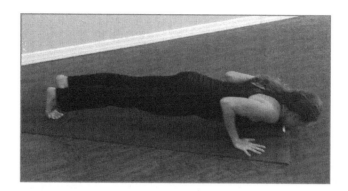

1. From table pose, widely spread your palms as if to suction the hand to the floor. Space your fingers while rooting from the hearth through the palm center and keeping your pointer finger's largest knuckle connected firmly.
2. Breathing into the core, visualize the kidney region inflating while keeping the shoulders engaged and heart softened towards the earth.
3. Keeping the shoulders over the wrist, begin to inch the knees back maintaining the core and kidney alignment.
4. On the inhale lift the knees from the floor and straighten the legs while having the bottom of the toes down, and heels directly up.
5. Lighten the posture by lifting in the core and extending forward through the crown of the head, and back through the heels. Press the thigh bones back into the hip sockets and up towards the sky.
6. Maintaining steady breath, use the exhale to slowly lower the straight horizontal body towards the floor making sure to tuck the elbows inward toward the ribs. The hips

do not sink before the rest of the body. If they do, release the knees towards the floor and continue to lower.
7. Hover above floor several inches at first then gradually lower without touching the floor. Gently hug the elbows in without losing the integrity of the hands.
8. Come out of the posture on an exhale by lowing to the ground gently or pressing the hands down to draw back up to plank.

11. Bhujangasana (Cobra)

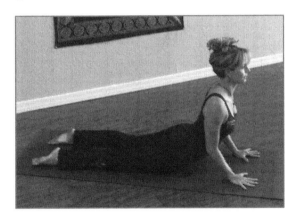

1. Laying with the front of the body on the floor, place the hands under the shoulders and roll the shoulders back and open. Keeping the shoulders and hands placed, press the extended legs through the feet.
2. Engage all toe tops on the floor evenly, while gently rolling the front of the thighs inward toward each other.
3. With the forehead on the floor, lift the navel and lower belly away from the floor while anchoring the tailbone down and rolling under.

4. Keeping the core engaged, tailbone rolling down, toes evenly pressing, and shoulders rolled back and open, begin to inhale the chest forward and slowly upward. IF there is any compression in the low back, return to the floor, work the core and tailbone again, then repeat slowly. If the low back compression still remains, ask for assistance.
5. Staying in the lifted chest cobra posture for several breaths, picture the front of the chest flowering open and the heat from the heart descending to the low hara.
6. Come out of the posture by exhaling back to the floor.

12. Balasana

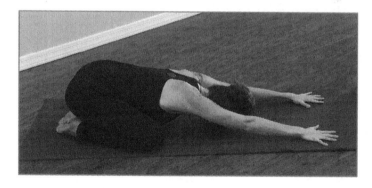

1. From table pose, inhale taking the knees as wide as the mat, and bring the toes together. Exhale drawing the hips back and over the heels as you slowly lower the chest towards the floor.
2. Stretch the arms forward onto the floor on the inhale, keeping the palms down and the arm bones lifting upward. The eyes of the elbows face each other with

engaged shoulder blades drawing down the back and towards the spine during the exhale.

3. Inhale to lengthen the spine and torso, exhale to roll the tailbone down towards the earth and lightly tucking under the pelvis.
4. Make sure to keep the tops of the shoulders broadening away from the neck, while keeping the hips back and sinking without dropping the active core or collapsing the kidney space.
5. Stay in the posture for several breaths allowing relaxation and a sense of calm to come over the body and self.
6. Inhale back up to table to come out of the posture.

13. Marjaryasana (Cat)

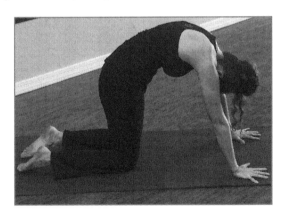

1. From a neutral spine in table pose, keep the quality of the hands and heart space as you inhale and begin to arch the spine convexly up towards the sky like a halloween cat tucking the tailbone under and the chin towards the chest. Exhale back to neutral.

2. Each moment in cat pose focuses on expanding the kidney space, activating the core, and lengthening the spine and side bodies.
3. Ultimately cat pose will alternate with cow pose.

Bitilasana (Cow)

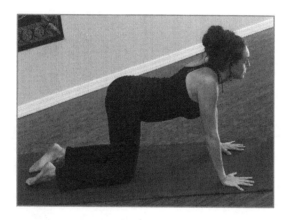

1. From table pose, keep the quality of the hands and shoulders. Exhale allowing the spine to descend into the body and creating a concave back. Draw the chin upward as if stretching a string connecting the chin and navel.
2. Engage the shoulder blades onto the back, melting the heart towards the floor in a broadening fashion.
3. To release the posture inhale back to a neutral spine.
4. Ultimately this posture alternates with cat pose.

14. Adho Mukha Svanasana/Cat Stretch

1. From table pose, begin to build the foundation of the posture by spreading and almost suctioning the hands to the mat while spacing the fingers widely. Structure the shoulders directly over the wrists and begin to soften the thoracic spine down towards the heart while drawing the shoulder blades down the back, engaging toward spine.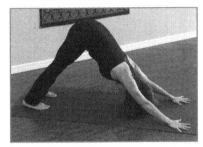

2. With the knees hip distance apart, curl the toes under and begin to lengthen the torso, being sure to keep the core engaged and tailbone drawing long and down the back of the legs. Extend the heart space forward with eyes between the hands and oppose with the side bodies becoming long.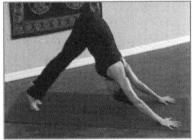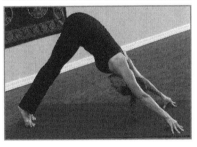

3. On an inhale slowly slide the hips back towards the heels, then begin to lift the hips and knees away from the floor while keeping the predominant amount of weight in the legs and out of the hands. Lift the buoyant hips up and back. Exhale the legs straight while working the heels towards the mat.

4. While in the posture, let the breath give life to the posture. Each inhale lightly bend the knees, lengthen the spine, and reach the hips up and back by lifting the core into the hips. Use the exhale to stay back into the legs and root the heels to the mat. Repeat for several breaths until in optimal position, which is held for a few more breaths.
5. To advance the posture, continue to cat stretch by raising onto the tips of the toes and if possible onto the fingertips.
6. Come out of the posture by exhaling the knees to the mat.

15. R Vasisthasana to Camatkarasana

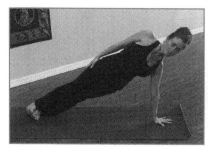 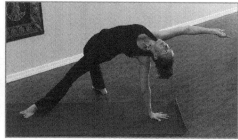

1. From plank pose, roll on the outside of the active right foot and transfer the weight to the right hand and foot.
2. Roll the body gently open so the chest faces the left side of mat while balancing on right outer foot and active right hand.
3. Let the body become buoyant by inhaling, engaging muscular action and lifting the right hip from the floor. While exhaling, extend equally through crown of head and feet.

4. Once steady, place the left hand on the left lifted hip. If steady there, advance by extending the left arm and hand actively into the air as if reaching to grasp something.
5. To move to camatkarasana, exhale to touch the left foot on the ground. Then begin to inhale to express the heart upward and the right arm opens and reaches slightly back to the right.
6. Limit the posture to skill level, and always come out if compression on lower back occurs.
7. Inhale back to side plank, and exhale to plank to come out of the posture. Repeat on other side.

16. R Tri Pada Adho Mukha Svanasana

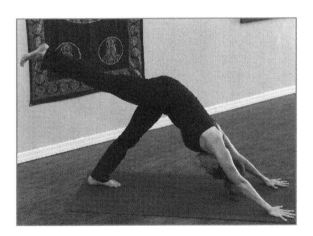

1. From downward dog, keep the action of the arms and expression of the hands as you begin to stabilize your right foot and inhale to lift the extended left leg.
2. In the same way and mind of the right heel rooting, continue to lift the left leg up. Exhale extending through the heel while keeping the pelvis lifted and level.

3. Maintaining the broadening of the ribcage forward, keep the leg lifted without twisting the torso or pelvis or collapsing the posture. Stay for several breaths.
4. Exhaling the left leg down to come out of the posture.
5. Repeat on other side.

17. L Vasisthasana to Camatkarasana

See instructions for Posture 15.

18. L Tri Pada Adho Mukha Svanasana

See instructions for Posture 16.

19. L Anjaneyasana

See instructions for Posture 6.

20. L Banarasana

See instructions for Posture 7.

21. L Utthan Pristhasana (Lizzard)

See instructions for Posture 8.

22. R Urdhva Prasarita Ekapadasana

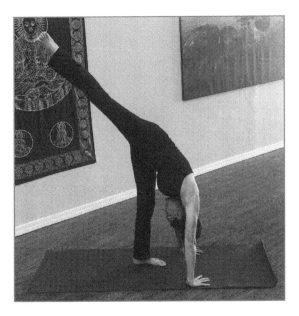

1. Standing split posture begins from uttanasana. First, implement the qualities of uttanasana.
2. Next, transfer the weight to the right leg as you begin to inhale and lift the left leg without turning the hip open.
3. Keeping that, exhale bringing expressive energy all the way up the left leg through the toes.
4. Use the inhalation to lengthen the spine, and the exhale to fold the face inward to the shin. The core inflates upward to the kidneys and lengthening will bow you closer as you hold behind the right ankle.
5. Repeat for several breaths.
6. Exhale the left leg down and rest a few breaths.

23. L Urdhva Prasarita Ekapadasana

See instructions for Posture 22.

24. Malasana

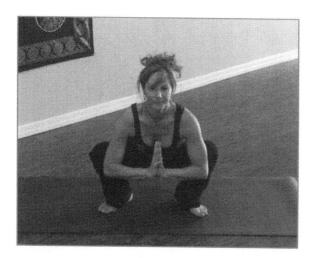

1. Squat with feet as close together as able, keeping heels on floor or on a folded blanket.
2. Keep the thighs outside the torso, allowing the torso to bow slightly forward between the legs.
3. Create isometric action between the elbows pressing inside the knees and the knees equally pressing back on the elbows while keeping a long spine and active tailbone.
4. Advance the posture by wrapping the arms around the front of the shins and clasping the heels with the hands.
5. Maintain the posture for several breaths, using the inhale to stand out of the posture.

25. Bakasana

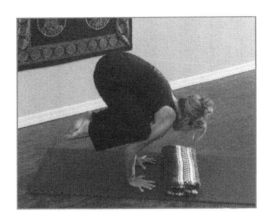

1. From uttanasana, bring your feet as close together as possible. Bend the knees and reach the hands forward in front of you about a foot or so.
2. Steady the palms on the ground by rooting all corners of the hands firmly onto the mat. Then widen the knees further apart than the hips.
3. On exhale begin to shift weight forward onto the balls of the feet and into the hands while keeping a lifted core.
4. Slide the inner knees up the outer biceps, inching towards the armpits yet keeping a grip of the inner knee on the outer arm with strong isometric action. Keeping this, move more weight into the toes and see if you can lift off the ground. Beginners should pause and work here until steady and confident.
5. To advance the posture, maintain a strong sense of core as you slowly transfer all the weight into the hands until the shoulders come a good bit forward of the hands.
6. Exhale out of the posture bringing the feet back to the earth.

26. Utkatasana

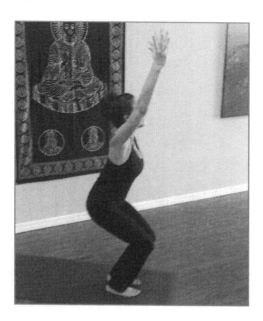

1. From tadasana, inhale and lift the arms up towards the sky keeping the palms facing each other or touching.
2. Exhale bending the knees deeply and bringing the thighs parallel to the floor or as close as parallel as possible.
3. Engage the shoulder blades onto the back while stabilizing with a rooted tailbone and under the pelvis.
4. Create an elongated torso drawing the sides long.
5. Take multiple breaths in the posture until inhaling back to tadasana.

27. Samastitihi

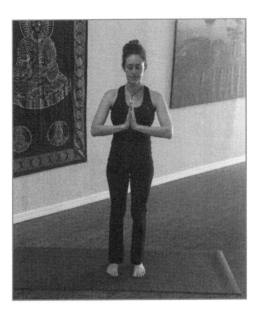

1. While inhaling, lift the crown of the head and lightly tuck the chin to lift the lower occipital ridge, then exhale and descend the tailbone down between the rooting legs and feet.
2. Lengthen the torso by extending the waist and releasing the chest open while keeping the pelvic floor level and heavy.
3. Inhale as the shoulders broaden down and away from the neck. Exhale and draw the bottom inner tips of the shoulder blades together and in towards the heart.
4. Lift the navel towards the spine and expand the kidneys.
5. Keeping legs weighted and engaged, inhale as you hug and wrap all of the muscles on the legs towards the bones of the legs, then exhale and extend the bones of the legs

into the earth as though they are a rooting tree while keeping the tailbone rooted.
6. The legs are straight yet knees are not locked. The thigh bones are turning inward as if corkscrewing the femur into the back of the hip socket. With each inhalation lengthen the torso. With each exhalation bow the torso over the legs.
7. Samatitihi joins the equally pressing palms at the lower heart space, symbolizing the right and left aspect of the body in harmony. Be still throughout, to find this moment, clear the past, and re-balance.

Section Two
28. R Alanasana (Crescent Lunge)

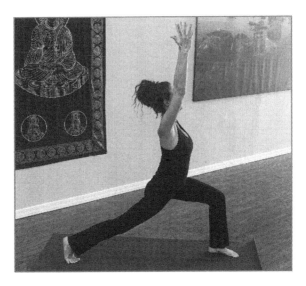

1. From downward dog, inhale lifting the right leg up and back, then exhale swinging the right leg (with control) forward between the hands coming into lunge pose.
2. Inhale curling the left toes under and lifting the left heel towards the sky. Exhale and steady the pose with muscular action of the legs.
3. Inhale drawing the arms over the head as if reaching for the sky, exhale and descend the shoulder blades down the back and inward towards spine. Palms face each other or are in namaste mudra.
4. Maintain a lifted and open heart space while holding the posture for several breaths.
5. Repeat on other side.

29. R Virabhadrasana I

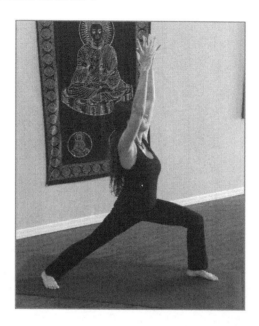

1. From lunge pose with right leg forward, exhale the left heel down with the foot open at a 45-degree angle. Inhale drawing up supportive prana from the earth, and exhale rooted action back into the earth.
2. Inhale and draw the arms over the head, fingers pointing up and palms facing each other. Exhale and descend the shoulders.
3. Maintain the posture by always keeping the front knee directly over the front ankle and never in front of the ankle while settling into the front leg yet rooting through the back heel. Keep thinner thighs active and lifting to support the femur bone.
4. While staying in the posture add awareness to both the tailbone and core, drawing up and back for support of the even pelvis, keeping the heart expanding and open.

5. Come out on the exhale by lowering the hands to the floor on either side of the right foot and returning to lunge.
6. Repeat on other side.

30. R Baddha Virabhadrasana

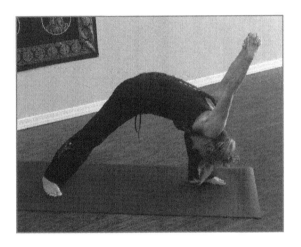

1. From Virabhadrasana I, bring the arms down behind the back and interlace the fingers. Inhale and roll the shoulders up, then exhale the shoulder blades down the back and towards the spine.
2. Maintaining a strong core and rooted tailbone, extend the spine on the inhale while opening the front heart space. On the exhale bow forward folding at the hips with a level pelvis. Allow the head to drop (unless you have high blood pressure) and draw the arms with interlaced fingers forward towards your head.
3. Remain in the posture for several breaths before inhaling to return to virabhadrasana I.
4. Repeat on other side.

31. Urdhva Mukha Svanasana

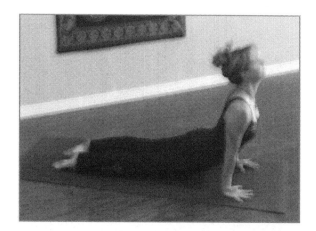

1. Start by laying belly down on the mat. Place the expanding hand outside the heart space by the shoulders.
2. Press all ten toenails onto the mat as you rotate the inner active thighs in towards the groin and back towards the sky.
3. Inhale pressing the tops of the feet down, while raising the upper torso, elevating the crown of the head as if being lifted at the top of the head. Exhale and settle the heart forward and open into the posture.
4. If there is any compression at the low back, come out immediately and try again or seek a professional to assist.
5. Come out of the posture on the exhale as you lower to the mat.

32. L Alanasana (Crescent Lunge)

See instructions for Posture 28.

33. L Virabhadrasana I

See instructions for Posture 29.

34. L Baddha Virabhadrasana

See instructions for Posture 30.

35. R Utthita Parsvakonasana

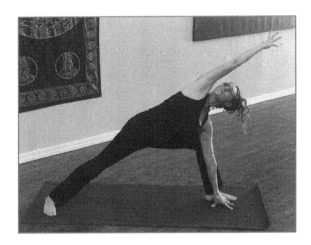

1. From lunge pose with the right foot forward roll the back left heel down to the mat with toes open. Create a straight line from the front heel to the back arch.
2. Bring the right hand gently without weight down next to the right foot.
3. Roll the torso open to the left as you extend the side bodies by lengthening from the iliac crest to the arm pits without crimping the shoulders around the neck. Inhale the left hand to the left hip, holding for a breath or so to stabilize the posture. Once you feel steady, draw the left arm over the left ear as you reach the left arm forward past the head.

4. Extend the back heel into the earth to oppose the reaching of the crown of the head.
5. Inhale the left rib cage up and expand ribs lightly with each breath in. On the exhale let go of unneeded tension.
6. Upon completion of the posture exhale the left hand to the floor and the left heel up towards the sky returning to lunge.
7. Repeat on other side.

36. R Virabhadrasana II

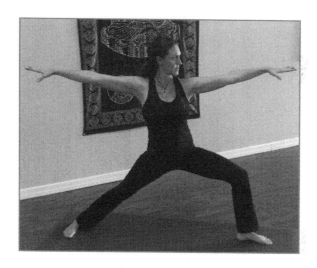

1. From extended side angle pose, root the active legs into the earth on the exhale, then on the inhale draw strength up from the earth through the core of your being as you raise the torso up to a vertical position.
2. As you rise to the posture, maintain a rooted tailbone, elongated spine, and a mindful core that expands the kidneys back.

3. Once the torso is vertical, extend the arms forward and back exhaling extension from the heart through the fingertips as you roll the shoulder blades down the back.
4. Maintain the posture with a light and lively lifted spirit through the crown of the head, long side bodies, weighted pelvis and strong inner thighs for several breaths.
5. Come out of the posture on the exhale by cartwheeling the arms to the earth with one hand on either side of the front foot, then lift the back heel to return to lunge.
6. Repeat on other side.

37. R Viparita Virabhadrasana I—Reverse Warrior

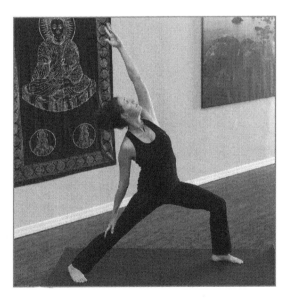

1. From warrior II, inhale lifting the front arm up, fingertips facing the sky and palm facing slightly back. Exhale to allow the back hand to touch the back thigh without weight or collapse of the long side bodies.

2. Keeping the qualities of warrior II, inhale the chest open and lifted, exhale the shoulders down the back away from the neck. Focus the eyes toward the hand in the air without scrunching the shoulders around the neck or losing length at the back of the neck. Maintain the posture for several breaths.
3. Inhale out of the posture to warrior II, then to the earth for lunge.
4. Repeat on other side.

38. R Trikonasana

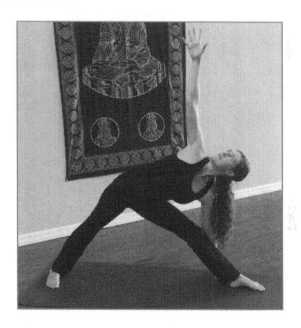

1. From extended side angle pose with right leg forward, place the right hand outside the right foot on the mat or block.
2. At first, bring the left hand to the left hip.

3. On the inhalation begin to straighten the front leg until straight with the knee unlocked. On the exhale, draw the right hip back and begin to create space in the side body between the hip and armpit without shrugging the shoulders around the neck.
4. Strengthen your resolve of the posture and activate the leg muscles to the bone, as the bone extends outward into the earth. Keeping this, roll the tailbone under and draw the core in and up.
5. Focus on lengthening the spine as you open the heart towards the side, keeping the shoulders stacked on top of the other. Keeping that position, turn the eyes to the heavens gazing past the top hand.
6. Inhale and hug into the posture, then exhale and expand outward in all directions. Repeat for several breaths, then exhale out of the posture by bending the front knee, cartwheeling the arms to the earth, and lifting the back heel returning to lunge.
7. Repeat on other side.

39. R Ardha Chandrasana

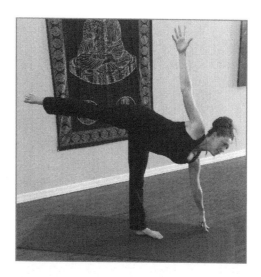

1. From triangle pose with right leg forward, keep all engaging and expanding qualities then bend the front right knee and reach the right hand forward about a foot, placing it either on the floor or a block.
2. Steady yourself as you transfer your weight forward to the right leg by slowly hopping the left foot forward and eventually lifting the left leg.
3. As you lift the rear left leg, be sure to expand both through the crown of the head, as well as back through the left foot.
4. Engage the core action to expand into the kidneys while anchoring the pose with the tailbone.
5. Inhale creating a lift along the left side body and inner left leg to lighten the posture, as if to draw the energy up from the earth through the standing leg and out all other peripheral directions such as the left hand, foot, side body, and head.

6. Mindfully keep the right hip drawing back so the right side body remains elongated. Remain for a few breaths.
7. Beginners may find confidence in this posture by practicing against the wall. Exhale out of the posture by releasing the left foot and hand to the floor in uttanasana.
8. Repeat other side.

40. R Ardha Chandra Chapasana

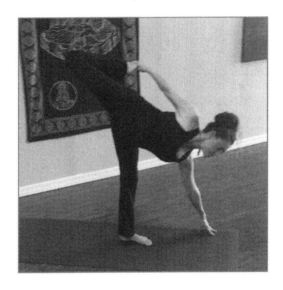

1. From ardha chandrasana posted on the right leg, steady yourself while keeping all points of awareness.
2. Begin bending the left knee towards the gluteus. Then after extending the left arm, circle the left arm around in front of the chest and continue the circle to the left toes.
3. With and engaged and well seated left shoulder, grasp the toes (or use the belt to do so).

4. Work in the posture for several breaths while keeping the side bodies long, the heart expanding forward, weight centered over right leg, active core, and tailbone anchored.
5. Inhale out of the posture by releasing the clasp slowly, extending to ardha chandrasana, and back to uttanasana.
6. Repeat on other side.

41. Throw a Ball

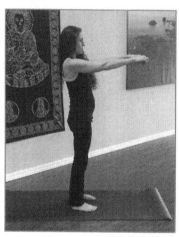 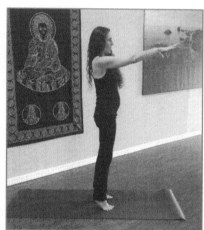

1. From tadasana, bring the arms forward, closed palms face down, and parallel to the floor with the wrist directly in front of the relaxed shoulders.
2. Inhale and lift up on the toes as you flick the fingers forward and out from under the tucked thumb. Exhale feet back to floor.
3. Repeat up to 300x's total.
4. Note that when doing multiple repetitions, the breath may not coordinate with movement.

42. Horse Stance

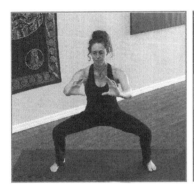 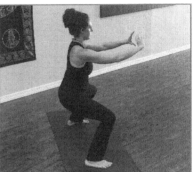

1. From tadasana, turn the toes out as far as your range allows, then keeping the toes out, turn the heels out as far as your range allows. From there repeat that action again until you are standing with feet about double hip distance apart.
2. Roll the tailbone lightly under until the pelvic floor is directly over the earth. Align the spine and back crown of the head over the tailbone.
3. Lift the front low belly below the navel up and in as if sucking in to zip up tight pants while making sure to spread the interior of the low belly towards each hip and kidneys.
4. Check that the knees are not in front of the toes, and the chest is not bowing forward.
5. Then on the exhale slowly bend the knees, keeping the alignments while sitting back into the hips and heels, yet keeping the toes gripping and pressure on the front balls of the feet.

6. Sink into the posture until you find your range limit. Stay there and breathe for several breaths, adding several breaths each day until able to hold for five minutes.
7. Ultimately the thighs will be parallel to the floor.
8. Inhale and straighten legs to standing to come out of posture.

43. Hold the Moon on a Golden Platter

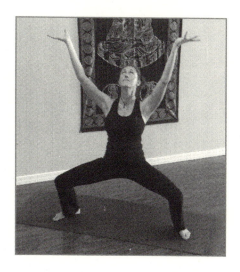

1. From horse stance, inhale and bring the palms face up and fingers pointed out, near the front outer shoulders.
2. Exhale to sink into horse stance while pressing the hands above the head as if holding a very heavy large platter.
3. Drop the shoulders, and imagine the weight of the platter sitting on the hips.
4. Keep the hands above the head, as you gently roll the heart open and upward towards the sky.
5. Remain in the posture for several breaths, and inhale to stand out of the pose, then exhale to release the arms.

44. L Utthita Parsvakonasana

See instructions for Posture 35.

45. L Virabhadrasana II

See instructions for Posture 36.

46. L Viparita Virabhadrasana—Reverse Warrior

See instructions for Posture 37.

47. L Trikonasana

See instructions for Posture 38.

48. L Ardha Chandrasana

See instructions for Posture 39.

49. L Ardha Chandra Chapasana

See instructions for Posture 40.

50. R Parivrtta Utkatasana

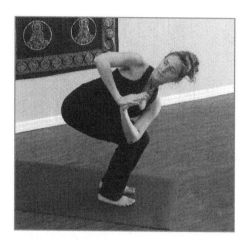

1. From chair pose, inhale and bring the hands to clasp palms or namaste mudra at the lower hearth center.
2. Exhale pressing the hands together evenly to give your self a sense of center. Do not allow the shoulders to come up.
3. Draw the side bodies long on the inhale, the core back, and the tailbone down on the exhale.
4. Bring your mind to the navel center and begin twisting left from there without loosening the hands centered at the sternum.
5. Twisting cautiously with a long torso, trying to bring your right elbow outside your left knee.
6. Connect the right elbow outside the left knee and create equal action of the right elbow and left thigh connecting.
7. Maintain the posture for several breaths, lengthening on the inhale and working the twist on the exhale.
8. Come out of the posture on the inhale returning to chair pose, then exhale to press the legs down and stand up.
9. Repeat on other side.

51. R Parivrtta Anjaneyasana

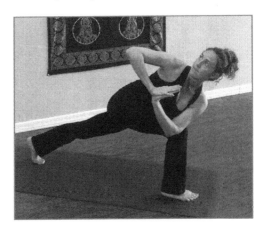

1. From lunge pose, inhale and bring the hands to clasp palms or namaste mudra the lower hearth center.
2. Exhale pressing the hands together evenly to give your self a sense of center. Do not allow the shoulders to come up.
3. Draw the side bodies long on the inhale, the core back, and the tailbone down on the exhale.
4. Bring your mind to the navel center and begin twisting left from there without loosening the hands centered at the sternum.
5. Twisting cautiously with a long torso, try to bring your right elbow outside your left knee.
6. Connect the right elbow outside the left knee and create equal action of the right elbow and left thigh connecting.
7. Maintain the posture for several breaths, lengthening on the inhale and working the twist on the exhale.
8. Come out of the posture on the inhale returning to lunge pose, then exhale to release the hands to the mat.
9. Repeat on other side.

52. Prasarita Padottanasana

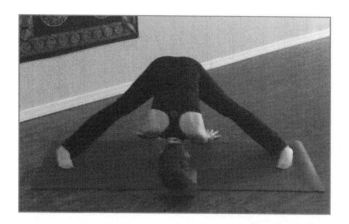

1. From tadasana, bring your hands to your hips and walk or jump the feet widely apart, turning the toes in ever so slightly.
2. Lengthen the torso up out of the settled pelvis with the inhale. On the exhale draw the shoulder blades onto the back to lift the heart and lightly tuck the chin to open the cervical vertebrae.
3. Inhale drawing the internal torso long, then on the exhale fold at the hips (not the waist) and bow forward slowly with an active core to protect the low back.
4. Slowly lower hands to the mat or blocks as you fold, keeping the inner thighs strong and lifted from the earth and outer feet and big toe anchored to the mat.
5. When you reach your forward bend depth or range, remain there for several breaths. If you are able and desire to go further in the pose, begin walking the hands through the legs and back behind you with the idea of bringing the crown of the head to the mat.

6. Remain in the posture for several breaths, using the inhale to extend, and the exhale to deepen the posture.
7. To come out of the posture, place the hands on the hips, inhale and bring the torso vertical while keeping a straight spine and strong core. Exhale to stand.

53. R Parivrtta Prasarita Padottanasana

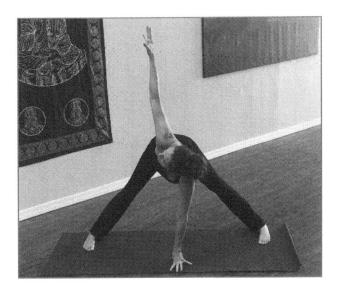

1. Keep all qualities of the standing wide angle forward bend, then place the right hand on the floor under the face with no pressure in the hand.
2. Inhale to bring the left hand to the left hip.
3. Exhale and begin to twist from below the navel to the left while maintaining a level pelvis.
4. Once stable in the posture you may extend the left arm up towards the sky.
5. Inhales are used to reach the hips back slightly, with the crown of the head forward and the spine lengthened.

6. The exhales strengthen the core and turn the torso deeper into the posture.
7. Come out of the posture by exhaling to return the torso to face the earth. Inhale the hands to the hips, and rise to a standing position.
8. Repeat on other side.

54. L Parivrtta Prasarita Padottanasana

See instructions for Posture 53.

55. L Parivrtta Utkastasana

See instructions for Posture 50.

56. L Parivrtta Anjaneyasana

See instructions for Posture 52.

57. Urdhva Hastasana/Double Palms

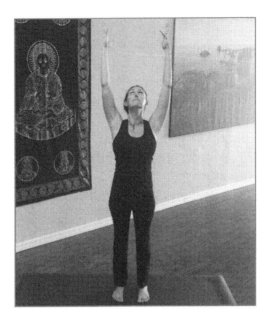

1. Stand with all of the qualities of tadasana.
2. Inhale and reach the arms forward and parallel to the earth. Exhale and pull the head of the arm bones back into the sockets.
3. Keeping that, inhale again and slowly begin to raise the arms towards the sky, stopping when you reach your range's edge.
4. The posture stretches in two directions, the inhale lengthens and the exhale roots.
5. Maintain the posture with focus on brightening the heart, and earthiness in the pelvis and legs.
6. Come out of the posture on the exhale by releasing the arms.

58. R Standing Crane

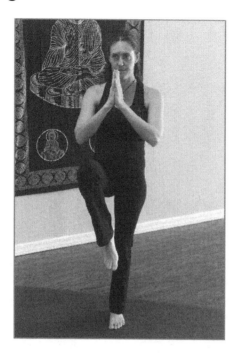

1. From tadasana, steady your weight over the unlocked right leg.
2. Press the hands together at the heart center to bring the mind from the periphery. Roll the tailbone lightly under and draw the widened core back towards the kidneys.
3. Lessen the weight on the left foot as you sink the weight into the right leg.
4. Inhale bending your left knee, drawing the leg up slowly as high as you are able.
5. Set your focus towards the floor and as you stabilize, slowly lift the gaze looking forward.
6. Exhale to come out of the posture.
7. Repeat on other side.

59. R Crane Points to 7 Star

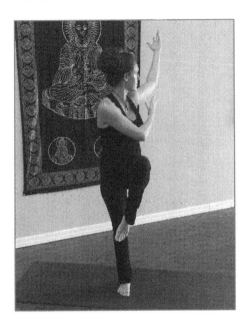

1. From standing crane, begin to reach the arms to the same side as your standing leg extends them up and back.
2. Do your best to draw the lifted leg up to eventually touch the bottom arm.
3. Once you feel steady, shift the gaze slowly back to look at the top back hand.
4. Come out by inhaling and turning the chest forward and exhaling the lifted leg back to the floor.
5. Repeat on other side.

60. R Hasta Padangusthasana

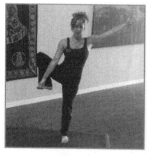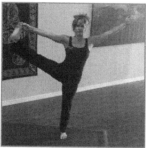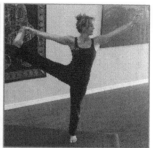

1. From tadasana transfer weight to the left leg and bend the right knee, lifting the leg and sinking your weight into the left leg. Lift the right leg until you can grasp the right foot.
2. Rotate the right knee up and around to open the right hip and set the femur bone back and down into the hip socket. Roll the outside of the right hip down so as to lengthen the side body between the right armpit and right hip.
3. Holding steady and grasping the right big toe with the first two fingers on the right hand, slowly extend the right leg up and out to the side as you extend your left hand up and out to the left for counter balance.
4. Maintain a rooted tailbone, long spine, lifted crown of the head and equal extension between the lifted foot and upward reaching hand.
5. Return to center and tadasana to come out of the posture.

61. R Vrksasana

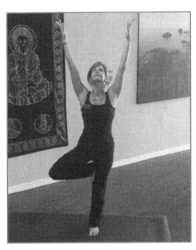 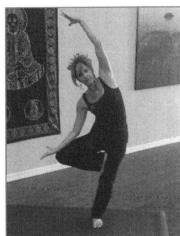

1. From tadasana bring your hands to namaste at the lower heart center and exhale rooted action into the earth. Inhale as you bring the hands up towards the sky, releasing the palms open and still facing each other while making sure the shoulders stay down and away from the neck.
2. Slowly transfer the weight to the left leg as you cautiously lift the right foot from the floor. Then open the right knee to slowly work the right foot up the inner left leg, avoiding pressure on the left knee until the right foot nestles into the inner left thigh. Hug the right foot and left thigh together.
3. Maintain a lengthened torso. Beginners stop here.
4. Should you feel ready to move on, lengthen the left side body to lean to the right without collapsing or compromising the right side body to arc over.
5. Inhale returning to center; exhale right foot to mat.
6. Rest then repeat.

62. R Virabhadrasana III

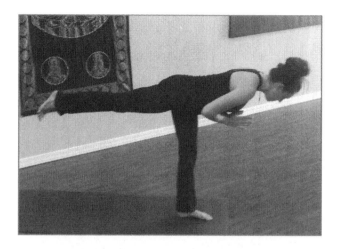

1. From virabhadrasana I, bend the front knee and slowly transfer the weight forward to stand on front leg. Inhale and lift the back leg while reaching forward through the crown of the head. Exhale and extend the body and mind in two directions: one through the crown of the head, and the other through the back lifted and engaged foot.
2. Support the posture by maintaining a lifted core and pressing up of the rear lifted leg's thigh bone into the hamstring or the sky while keeping the pelvis level.
3. The rear lifted toes should all point to the mat, and the hands may stay at the heart center in namaste mudra, or extend forward as though pretending to fly.
4. Each inhalation lifts the body, and each exhalation extends the body. Try practicing this pose at the wall to build confidence.
5. Remain in the posture for several breaths before inhaling and returning to tadasana or virabhadrasana I.
6. Repeat on other side.

63. R Natarajasana

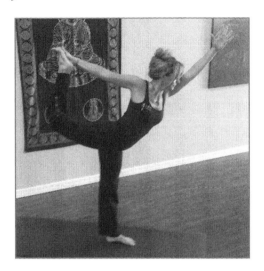

1. From tadasana, slowly transfer all of the weight into the left leg. Then steadily bend the right knee to bring the right foot towards the buttox.
2. Roll the right shoulder back and into the socket then reach for the right foot and clasp the inner ball of the foot.
3. Extend the left arm out and forward at an upward 45-degree angle to offer as a counter balance.
4. Once you feel steady in this position, slowly bow the torso forward creating a bow-like posture. Cautiously lengthen the right thigh and lift the right foot higher in the air.
5. Beginner suggestion is to use a looped strap to hold the right foot.
6. Inhale to center, exhale to standing to come out of the posture.
7. Repeat on other side.

64. R Garudasana

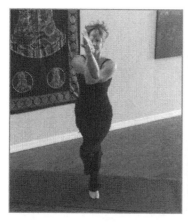 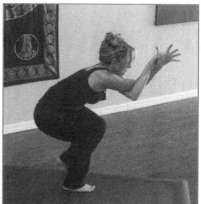

1. From tadasana, transfer all the weight over the right leg and steady all four corners of the left foot onto the ground.
2. Slowly take the left leg and cross it over the right thigh, doing your best to hug the outer left shin alongside the outer right shin. If flexibility allows, hook the left foot behind the right shin.
3. Next, take the left arm under the right arm, hooking at the elbows, and cross the wrist over again if able. Hug the engaged arms and hands together.
4. Once steady in pose, bend the right knee deeper, gently bowing forward and reaching arms forward while seating back the hips.
5. Inhale to unwind the posture and stand.
6. Repeat on other side.

65. L Standing Crane

See instructions for Posture 58.

66. L Crane Points to 7 Star

See instructions for Posture 59.

67. L Hasta Padangusthasana

See instructions for Posture 60.

68. L Vrksasana

See instructions for Posture 61.

69. L Virabhadrasana III

See instructions for Posture 62.

70. L Natarajasana

See instructions for Posture 63.

71. L Garudasana

See instructions for Posture 64.

Section Three
72. Moving 8 Vessels: 7 Stars Press Earth

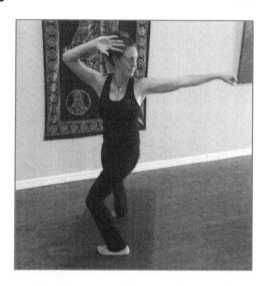

1. From tadasana, transfer all of the weight into the bent left leg, being sure to keep the left knee aligned with the left toes and not reaching forward over them.
2. From the uppermost right thigh rotate the entire right leg inward so the right foot is 45 degrees inward and the right toes point at the left toes.
3. Strengthen the inside of the right leg as if to lift the inner groin while keeping the tailbone rooted.
4. Then twisting from the waist (not hips or knees) create an upward lift through the torso and chest to turn towards the left leg, trying to line up the sternum with the left heel.
5. Draw the shoulders down the back as you reach the left arm with a robins egg fist out towards the side, keeping the arm perpendicular to the torso and parallel to the

floor, then draw the bent right arm up with the palm facing outward in front of the forehead.
6. Inhale to center to come out of the posture.
7. Repeat on other side.

73. Divide Heaven and Earth

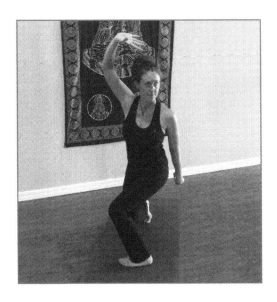

1. From 7 star stance posted on the left leg, lift the right heel while bending the knee to point at the ground.
2. Bring the left hand in cranes beak mudra down by the left hip and point it behind you to stretch the ligaments.
3. Inhale to center.
4. Repeat on other side.

74. Stand in Ba Pull Bow Shoot Arrow

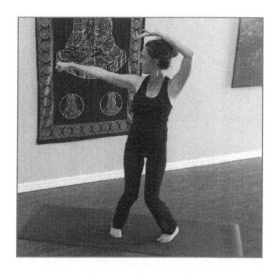

1. From tadasana walk the heels open to a 45-degree angle, allowing the knees to turn in, yet not collapse.
2. Extend the right arm outward with a robins egg fist, and the left arm bent over the head with palm up and relaxed shoulders.
3. Eyes focus down the right hand
4. Return to center and repeat on other side.

75. Twisted Stance to Push Two Poles

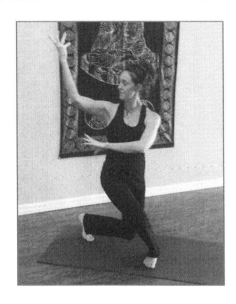

1. From tadasana, bring all your weight over the left leg. With caution step the empty right foot behind, placing the toes down and the heel pointing directly up.
2. Work the weight to an even pressure, eventually sinking the left knee to hover about a fist's distance above the floor. Turn the torso from the navel up on the exhale.
3. Bring the bent left arm across the body while turning the hand slightly as if tightening a jar.
4. The right arm bends reaching in the air as if turning in a light bulb. Make sure to keep the shoulders relaxed.
5. Inhale to center to come out of the posture.
6. Repeat on other side.

76. Crescent Moon

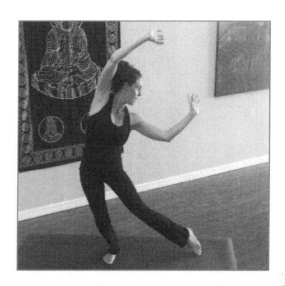

1. From tadasana stabilize the weight over the right leg then slowly reach the empty left toes as far out to the side as possible.
2. Lengthen the right side body as you raise your right arm up over the head, palm up and shoulder descending.
3. Reach the left arm out towards the side, palm up. Picture holding a stick in the hands. Focus the gaze towards the left hand.
4. Inhale to center to come out of the pose.
5. Repeat on other side.

77. Ride the Tiger

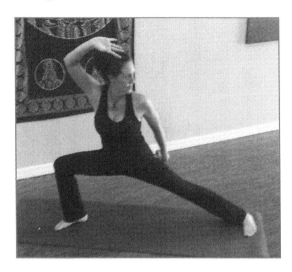

1. From horse stance, transfer the weight to the left leg to turn the right foot open to a 45-degree angle.
2. Then transfer the weight to the right leg to stretch the left leg back. Finally, settle the weight between the legs with the focus pressing down the left heel.
3. Extend a cranes beak left hand back around the left hip, and keep the right arm bent over the head, palm up with relaxed shoulder.
4. Keep the chest upright, then set the gaze over the left shoulder.
5. Inhale to center and work your way out of the posture and back to horse stance.
6. Repeat on other side.

78. Natural Palm Points to 7 Stars

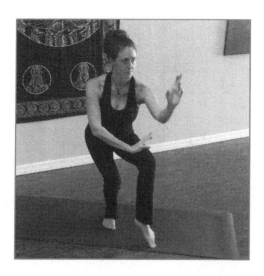

1. From ba stance, transfer the weight over the right bent right leg, keeping the knee from collapsing. Slowly extend the bent and empty right foot forward, touching only the tip of the toes to the floor.
2. Sit back with the hips while reaching forward with the chest and keeping shoulders relaxed.
3. Creating natural palms with both hands, reach the bent left arm forward with middle finger facing up, and the left bent arm slightly forward and middle finger pointing at the left elbow.
4. Inhale back to center
5. Repeat on other side.

79. Gather the Sun to Press the Earth

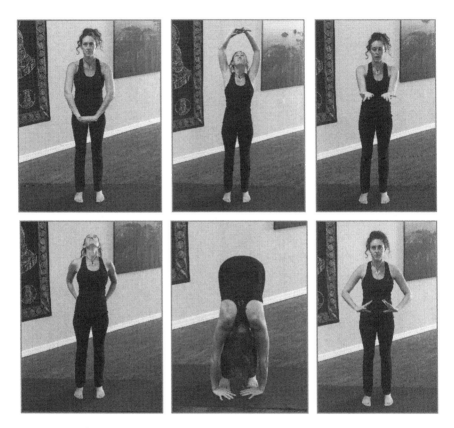

1. Start from tadasana, hands palms down below navel/low hara. Inhale and circle arms open towards sky, as you roll the sternum up towards the sky.
2. Bring the hands to the low back at the kidney space. Lift the chin looking up and exhale.
3. Inhale bowing forward at the hips (not waist) reaching for the floor. Hands go down the back of the legs to the toes then to the floor.
4. Bring the hands to the inner ankle and inhale as you roll the spine up, lightly rubbing the hands along the inner leg as you stand.

5. Exhale descending the hands from the sternum to below the navel to settle the prana into the low hara.
6. Repeat 3–5 more times.

80. Taoist Horse Stance

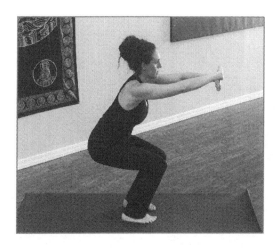

1. From tadasana, allow the gripping feet to be outer hip distance apart. Begin to lengthen the spine, tuck the chin to open the cervical vertebrae, make sure to root the tailbone, and broaden the core muscles back.
2. Extend the hands in front of the face, palms facing out with right palm on top of left palm. Set your drishti or gaze directly over the right pinky finger.
3. On the exhale, set your resolve and begin to bend the knees, syncing the hips back and down to bring yourself to a seated-like posture with thighs becoming parallel to the floor. Beginners start with less of a bend in the knees, and advance the posture until it becomes thighs parallel.
4. Hold the posture up to five minutes.
5. Inhale to stand and come out of the posture.

81. R Eka Pada Rajakapotasana Rising Up

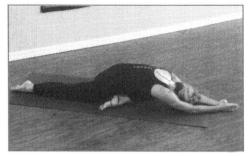
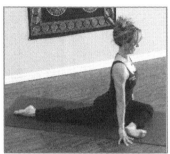
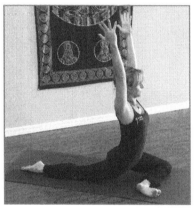
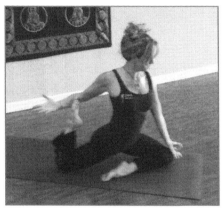

1. From tabletop posture, inhale and inch the left knee forward, as you inch the right knee back.
2. Swing the left foot inside towards the right hip. Beginners start with the foot tucked back towards the hip. Advanced posture, bring the left foot forward making the left shin perpendicular to the mat.
3. Keep an engaged tailbone, strong core pulling back towards the kidneys, and muscular action in the legs as you reach the right leg back and straight. Keep the right toes all facing the mat and roll the right inner thigh inward towards the groin.

4. For the forward fold action of this posture, exhale and lower the elbows to the mat down in front of the left leg, allowing the torso to bow forward. You can bring the forehead to the floor if flexibility allows. Make sure the core stays lifted and strong and there is no collapse in the mid body.
5. For the heart opening action, keep the legs engaged, pressing the left outer shin to the floor, rolling in the right thigh bone, and pressing the right shin bone and toe tops to the earth. With a strong core and rooted tailbone, inhale and lengthen the torso vertically, bringing the crown of the head to face the ceiling with a slightly tucked chin. Fingertips can stay on the floor on either side of the mat or body, or inhale and draw them up over the head towards the ceiling if the core feels strong enough.
6. In the heart opening portion of the posture, keep the shoulder blades engaged to the back tops of the shoulders rolling down the back while broadening open the front of the heart.
7. Working towards full king pigeon pose, bend the right knee, drawing the heel towards the hip. Hook the active foot into the crook of the right elbow. Hug the inner thighs together to create a lifted posture. Work to maintain all previous points of alignment.
8. Maintain the posture in a forward fold or heart opening focus for several breaths. Slowly work your way out of the posture and back to tabletop pose.
9. Repeat on other side.

82. R Eka Pada Rajakapotasana w/Fold

See instructions 1–4 of Posture 81.

83. L Eka Pada Rajakapotasana Rising Up

See instructions for Posture 81.

84. L Eka Pada Rajakapotasana w/Fold

See instructions 1–4 of Posture 81.

85. Ustrasana

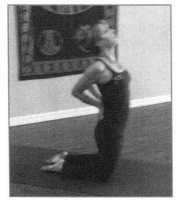
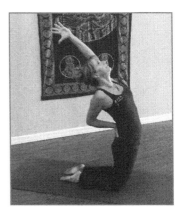
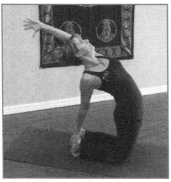
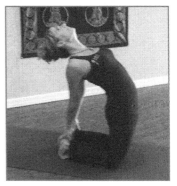

1. From a kneeling posture with shins and toe tops on the floor, and the torso vertical, begin to draw the arms

around behind the back. Do this by first moving the right arm out in front of you on the inhale. Then exhale while circling the arm above and behind you, bringing it to the low back, palm facing the back of the body. Fingertips may point as shown, but ideally should point up the back with the heel of the hand resting on the top of the gluteus. Repeat with left arm.
2. Once you have both hands on the low back between the kidneys and gluteus, engage the shoulder blades onto the back and draw the elbows towards each other to create a strong back body and a broadening and open heart space.
3. Create good quality action in the legs by turning the inner thighs in towards the groin, but make sure to maintain space between the uppermost part of the inner thigh, pushing the femur bones outwards in the hip sockets. Once you have done this, engage the tailbone rooting it down. Check the quality of the core by lifting from the lowest part of the low hara up to the navel and back towards the kidney space.
4. Keeping this, you may advance the posture slowly and cautiously. Try reaching one arm up behind you with the arm straight and palm facing inward, fingertips reaching. Then try to bring one hand at a time to the heel with the toes curled under.
5. Inhale slowly out of the posture then exhale to table.

86. Virasana

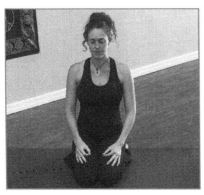 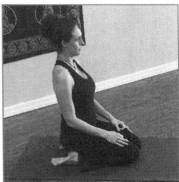

1. Start your posture in a kneeling position with a couple of blocks and/or a blanket next to you.
2. Begin by bringing the knees towards each other and the feet apart wider than the hips. At first take a block or two and put them between the ankles underneath the hips. Before you sit down, take hold of the right calf muscle and roll it open, moving it out to the side and away from the body. Repeat with the left calf muscle.
3. Then with a long spine, rooted tailbone, and gently engaged core, begin to sit the hips down on the blocks. If the posture is difficult add a blanket between the thighs and calves. If the posture is needing more challenge, remove one block at a time. Eventually your hips will sit on the floor between the ankles. Make sure to keep the tops of the feet on the mat as well as all ten toenails, especially the pinky toenails. Rest the hands on the legs.
4. Come out of the posture by pressing hands into the mat, lifting the hips, and sitting behind your feet as you bring the legs out straight in front of you.

87. Setu Bandha Sarvangasana

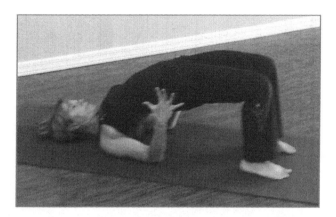

1. From a reclined posture with knees bent and feet on the floor about ten inches from the hips, begin the posture by bringing the shoulder blades towards each other on the back to engage a heart lifting space. Tuck the chin lightly to align the cervical vertebrae.
2. Next, with feet firmly planted on the ground, knees directly over the ankles, begin relaxing inner groin and thighs as if allowing them to melt towards the floor. Bring mindfulness to the tailbone, rooting it down towards the back of the knees while also broadening the core muscles inside the pelvic girdle.
3. Once these principles are in place, inhale pressing feet down to slowly raise the hips, and curl the chest forward and up as if bringing it over the neck towards the face. Lift the hips cautiously, ceasing the posture if there is any spinal discomfort. Hands may lie flat, palms down on ground with arms straight, or bent with elbows and fingers pointed towards the celling. Some enjoy supporting the hips with the hands.

4. Be sure the knees do not float outwards. They should stay directly over the ankles. Sometimes it's useful to place a block between the knees to press the legs to the block for good alignment.
5. If you are new to yoga or this posture, try starting by placing a block under the slightly lifted hips. Then allow the body to rest on the block for support while working the other points of alignment.

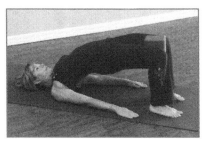 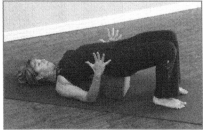

6. Come out of the posture by releasing the hips to the floor and allowing the inner knees to rest together.

88. Salamba Sarvangasana

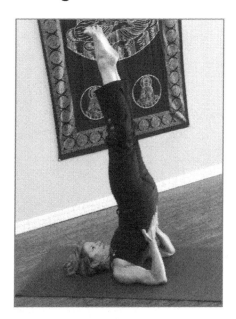

1. Starting from the same base is said to bond a sovereign gossen or bridge pose. Begin lying on your back with knees bent, feet about ten inches from the hips. Again begin to draw the shoulder blades onto the back working the elbows towards each other behind the back. Tuck the chin lightly to lengthen the cervical vertebrae.
2. Pressing the feet to the floor, keeping the knees sturdy over the ankles, and inner thighs relaxed with broadened core, inhale to begin lifting the hips cautiously from the floor.
3. Try to work the hips high enough to bring the hands under the hips and very low back. Begin working the heels closer to the heart space, as the heart space continues to expand up and forward as if drawing over the neck and face.

1. On the inhale begin to lift one leg straight at a time, until you can lift both legs directly up. Strengthen your resolve and the core, pulling the torso directly vertical over the shoulders and legs directly over the torso.
2. Shoulder stands being the mother of all postures presses on the fibroid glands in the throat space, making this a cleansing posture.
3. Beginners are encouraged to take blocks under the hips from the extended bridge pose, keeping the heart space lifting, active core, then lift one leg at a time while maintaining hips resting on one or two blocks. The effectiveness of the posture can still be found with hips on blocks, legs directly in the air, heart drawing forward, chin tucked and light pressure on the thyroid in the neck.
4. Advancing the posture turns into plow pose where one would keep the hips over the shoulders and begin to actively bring the legs to the floor, toes behind the head, and using core strength to lift the legs vertical once again.
5. Come out of the posture rolling the spine down, bending the knees into the chest and coming down very slowly.
6. This posture, although level one, can be considered an intermediate and advanced posture. Beginners are advised to work with blocks under the hips, a folded blanket under the shoulders to the elbows, and always under the supervision of a trained instructor.

89. R Sucirandrasana

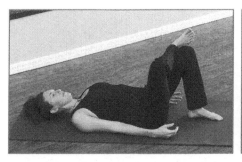 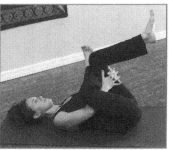

1. From a reclined position, bend the knees, placing the feet flat on the floor about ten inches from the hips.
2. After engaging the shoulder blades onto the back, lightly tucking the chin to elongate the back of the neck, take the right ankle with active foot crossing over the left thigh just below the left knee. Be sure to keep the right knee and ankle in a straight line.
3. While keeping the side bodies long, bring the left thigh towards the body by either interlacing the fingers behind the mid thigh, or using a strap to hold behind the thigh and bring it close to the body. Make sure the left foot stays active.
4. Use the right elbow to wedge the right thigh away while drawing the left thigh inwards.
5. Maintain the posture for several breaths before releasing the left foot to floor, then right foot to floor.
6. Repeat other side.

90. R Agnistmbhasana

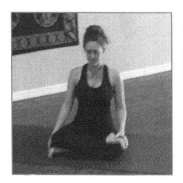 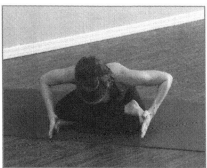

1. Begin in an easy seated posture on the mat or a folded blanket. Draw the flesh of the buttocks back and apart, root the tailbone, lengthen the torso, tuck the chin, and lift the crown of the head.
2. Start by bringing the right knee into the crook of the right elbow and holding the right foot with the left hand, making a baby cradle for the right leg. Then slightly bring the right ankle over the left knee, sliding the ankle slightly past the knee and keeping the right foot active while keeping the right shin parallel to the front of the hips.
3. If you are able to move on in the posture, begin to inch the left foot away from the groin and under the right knee. Make sure the left foot is active, as if the outer foot is karate chopping the floor. The toes of both feet are drawing slightly back towards each other. Keep the ankles straight and without crease on either side to the ankles.
4. If able to go to the next step of the pose, place the palms of the hands on the balls of the feet and create isometric action between the pushing of the balls of the feet and the pressure of the hands. Lengthen the torso up out of the

pelvis on the inhalation, and on the exhalation begin to bow forward over the legs.
5. To come out of the posture inhale the torso up and exhale releasing the left foot back towards the groin and the right foot off the left leg.
6. Repeat on other side.

91. R Gomukhasana

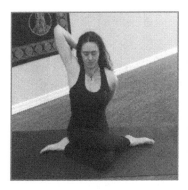 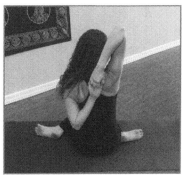

1. Sit either on the floor or mat with the legs straight out in front of you. Bend the left knee and draw the left foot towards the outer right hip. Then bend the right knee drawing the right foot to the out left hip.
2. Lengthen the torso upright, drop the shoulders, relax the chin down, and lift the inner crown of the head.
3. Draw the right arm forward with pinky finger pointed down and muscles that hug to the bones. Inhale the arm straight up. Once vertical, bend the right elbow to bring the tips of the fingers towards the thoracic spine. Next bring the left hand to the left hip, then slowly draw the left hand behind you with the back of hand facing the back itself.

1. Slowly slide the hands towards each other with caution until able to grasp fingers. Use a strap if needed to close the gap. Remain mindful to keep shoulders down and broadening away from neck. Do not overextend the arms to complete the pose.
2. Inhale and release the arms and exhale to straighten the legs one at a time.
3. Repeat on other side

92. L Sucirandhrasana

See instructions for Posture 89.

93. L Agnistambhasana

See instructions for Posture 90.

94. L Gomukhasana

See instructions for Posture 91.

95. Navasana

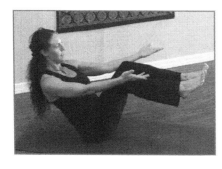 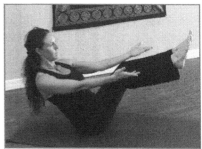

1. From dandasana, lift up the sternum and lengthen the torso out of the pelvic region. Spread the core wide and strong with letting it bulge.

2. After drawing the flesh of the buttocks back and apart, rest on the sits bones and tailbone.
3. Slowly begin to bend the knees bringing the shins up with active feet. At first, aim for getting the shins parallel to the mat. Then, if possible, begin to lift the shins higher, to a full straight leg extension if possible.
4. Maintain posture for several breaths.
5. Exhale out of the posture, bringing the feet to the floor, crossing the legs lightly, and folding gently to release.

96. Dandasana

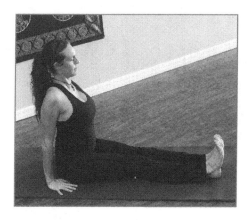

1. From a seated position with the hips on the floor or a folded blanket, begin by stretching the legs out forward together in front of you. Press the rolling inward and pulling back thigh bones into the floor while gently pulling back the active toes and gripping lightly with the heels.
2. Create a lifting core that pulls up the lower belly and draws it back through the navel towards the kidneys. Bring length to the torso and spine, with buoyancy

at the crown of the head and a slightly tucked chin so as to open the back of the neck. Draw the shoulder blades together towards the spine and down the back to create the open heart space.

1. Place the hands palms down on the mat, outside the hips.
2. Maintain the posture for several breaths, working extension-like movements on the inhale, and hugging into the core of the body and self on the exhale.

97. Paschimottanasana

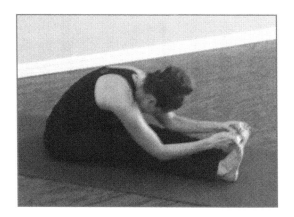

1. From dandasana, keep all points of alignment as you inhale the arms up towards the sky. With engaged core, begin to exhale a long torso forward over the thighs while reaching for the toes.
2. Beginners often enjoy sitting on a folded blanket and start by reaching for the calves, then working their way to a deeper posture.
3. Eventually, one is able to hold the toes or soles of the feet, with torso laid long over the legs.

4. Be sure to keep the shoulders broadened away from the neck.
5. Inhale length; exhale and fold.
6. Maintain posture for several breaths, working your way to five minutes.

98. R Marichyasana

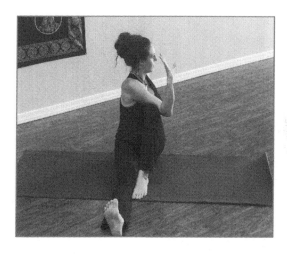

1. From dandasana, bend the left knee while bringing the left foot flat on the floor next to the right knee.
2. Inhale lengthening the spine as you lift from inside the crown of the head, then begin to slowly draw into the back body while keeping the chin level or ever so slightly tucked.
3. On the exhale draw the navel deeply towards the spine and begin to twist from the core towards the left leg without slouching the chest down. Lift the chest instead.
4. Each inhalation will lengthen the posture, each exhalation will enhance the twisting.

5. Inhale to center and come out of the posture, returning the left leg straight.
6. Repeat on other side.

99. L Marichyasana

See instructions for Posture 98.

100. R Janu Sirsasana Fold

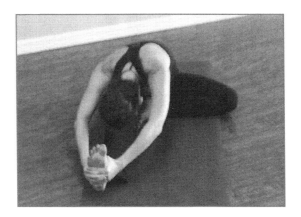

1. From a seated position, bring the right leg straight forward into a mild V. Tuck in the left heel towards the groin. Find a good seat, leveling the sitz bones onto the mat or a folded blanket.
2. Lengthen the torso, lifting the ribs away from the pelvis, while allowing the pelvis to remain earthy and rooted along with the tailbone.
3. Draw the shoulders back and down the back of the body, to broaden them away from the neck. With a lightly tucked chin, allow a lifted feeling through the inside crown of the head.

4. To begin the fold, lengthen the torso, root the pelvis, press the right thigh bone down and keep the right foot active with toes pointing up to the ceiling, and toes slightly drawn towards the body. Inhale lengthen, then exhale drawing the core wide and back to allow the torso to fold over the right leg. Bring the hands down the right leg, holding the shin or the feet. Beginners can use a strap around the foot to help draw the torso forward. Maintain the posture for several breaths, using the inhale to lengthen and the exhale to deepen the fold.
5. Come out of the posture by inhaling the torso back up and bending in the right knee.
6. Repeat on other side.

101. R Parivrtta Janu Sirsasana

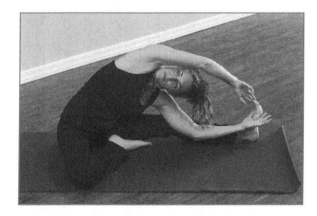

1. For the twist, start with the same base posture, seated with the right leg stretched forward and the left foot bent in towards the groin. Make sure to level the pelvis, lengthen the torso, tuck the chin, and lift the crown of the head.

2. Next, lifting the ribs lightly, turn the upper torso towards the left slightly. Place the right hand inside the right knee making sure to keep the right side body long between the hip and the armpit. Inhale for the length, then on the exhale slide the right hand towards the right foot. Then inhale the left arm up towards the sky, and exhale leaving the torso over the right leg reaching the left arm towards the right foot. The torso will be slightly turned towards the left side. Work the posture using the inhalation to create link, and the exhalation to twist and fold. Be sure to twist from the naval, and keep the side bodies long.
3. To come out of the posture, inhale the torso vertical, and exhale folding in the right leg.
4. Repeat on other side.

102. L Janu Sirsasana Fold

See instructions for Posture 100.

103. L Parivrtta Janu Sirsasana

See instructions for Posture 101.

104. Upavistha Konasana

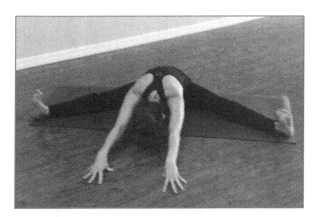

1. From a seated position, extend the legs open and out as far as possible without harming the body. It is often useful to sit on a folded blanket.
2. Upon extending the legs, make sure to keep the feet upright, heels lightly gripping the mat and active toes pointed towards the ceiling.
3. Press the thigh bones into the mat without over pressing the back of the knee. Keep the thigh bones rolling open, grounding the tailbone. Take hold of the flesh of the buttocks and pull it back and apart to allow a greater range of motion when bowing forward and to ease the seated posture.
4. Once you have established a good seat, inhale to lengthen the spine and engage the shoulder blades onto the back. Then to fold, exhale and begin rolling the pelvic floor forward towards the mat while keeping the torso long and mostly straight. The fold will happen at the hip/thigh crease and not the waist.

5. Each inhalation will lengthen the posture; each exhalation will fold the posture deeper.
6. Come to a place in the posture at the beginning edge of discomfort and reside there for multiple breaths. Deep stretching classes hold this posture three to five minutes.
7. Come out of the posture by inhaling the torso vertical, and exhaling the legs together.

105. Baddha Konasana

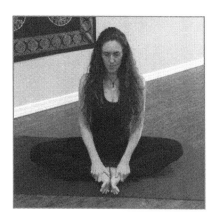

1. From a seated position either on the floor or on folded blanket(s), rest most of the weight on the sitz bones, rooting the tailbone and expanding the kidney space.
2. Bring the soles of the feet together, with an activeness throughout the legs and ankles to the toes.
3. Grasp the ankles, and draw the chest lightly forward and up, lifting the upper torso out of the lower heavy pelvis. Lightly anchor the chin while lifting inside the crown of the head, being sure to keep the shoulders down and broadened away from the neck.

4. Should the posture need more, begin the forward bend by lengthening the spine, then folding forward past the feet while maintaining an active core.
5. Inhale to rise. Exhale legs straight to come out of the posture.

106. Seated Holding a Golden Qi Ball Breathing/ Heal Sounds

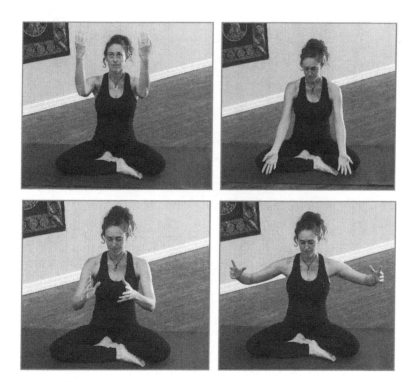

1. From siddhasana, slowly inhale the hands up in front of the body, palms facing in and fingers up.
2. Exhale fully and somewhat quickly as the hands fall to the front of the knees. If tendons are in good condition,

a small flick of the arms and wrist allows prana to better flow into the hands.
3. Inhale circling the arms open to chest height and palms facing each other.
4. Without breath, press the hands together as if there were tension and pressure to compress an object between the hands. Eventually the sensation of two magnets opposing each other in the palms becomes present.
5. Exhale allowing the hands to come together as if the magnets had flipped and are being drawn together.
6. Repeat 3–5 times.

107. Siddhasana w/Infinity Mudra

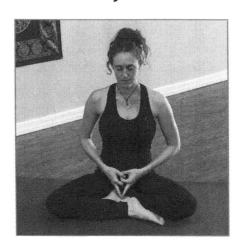

1. Fold in the legs, bringing one foot as close to the groin as possible and the other directly in front of the other. Often it is useful to sit slightly elevated on a block or folded blanket.
2. Create the infinity mudra by touching the tips of the thumbs and first fingers together, then interlacing the

looped fingers. Connect the tips of the middle fingers together, then the ring and pinky fingers.
3. Lightly place the hands in front of the low hara, looped fingers forward, and straight fingers pointed downward.
4. Sitting with a long spine, lifted crown of head, slightly tucked chin, relaxed shoulders, and open chest, begin your pranayama with focus on descending heat into the hara behind the hands.
5. It is often useful to focus the gaze behind closed eyelids to keep the eyes from wandering and stirring the mind.
6. Maintain the posture for three to five minutes, slowly increasing the length.

108. Savasana

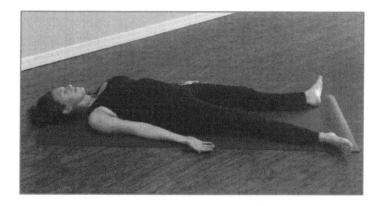

1. Lie down on your back, aligning yourself with the mat. Take the feet as wide as the mat and engage the shoulder blades onto the back, relaxing the palms face up. Tuck the chin slightly to elongate the neck.
2. Envision the chest relaxing open like butter in a warm pan.

3. Savasana is the hardest posture. The physical ease increases the difficulty to focus on the present moment. Often the seeker wanders into sleep or an unconscious state of mind.
4. Savasana invites one to stay present yet in a fully relaxed state.
5. Remember here that you are not your thoughts, not your emotions, and not your body.
6. Remain in the posture without commanding the breath for several minutes.
7. To come out of the posture, first take a few deep breaths, then while inhaling, slowly move the hands, feet, and head in a gentle rocking manner.
8. Inhale the knees to the chest, hugging them in towards the body. Rock gently side to side until you eventually roll to your right side in a fetal position.
9. After a few breaths, rise to seated posture by using your arms to push yourself up.
10. Remain in a seated posture for a moment or so, settling into the relaxation. Remember the feeling, and that you can return to it when desired.
11. Close your practice with gratitude for having the opportunity to cultivate.

Part 11

Pranayama
(Qi Gong Breath Work)

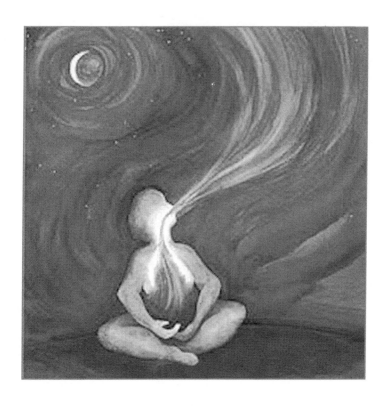

Pranayama (Qi Breathing)

Life starts and ends by taking a breath and it is obvious that we should fill our lives with good breathing habits. One teacher said, "If you knew you had a finite amount of breaths in this life, how would you use them? Would they be short and quick? Or long and deep?"

Our bodies need a lot of oxygen to function properly and to help discard waste products like carbon monoxide. Every cell in the body actually needs lots of oxygen. Today many people are conscious about what they drink and what they eat, but very few think about how they breathe!

Breathing affects the whole body. It affects the nervous system, the heart, the digestive system, muscles, sleep, energy levels, concentration, memory and much more. Breathing is also our largest system for waste removal. Seventy percent of the waste products produced in our body are supposed to be removed via breathing, 20 percent are removed via the skin and only 10 percent should remain for the kidneys and the digestive system to eliminate. We not only breathe in oxygen but also life energy (qi, or ki in Japan, and prana).

The majority of people only use chest breathing. This type of breathing is easily affected; it becomes easily restrained or blocked. People who use chest breathing take less effective breaths and, as a consequence, receive less oxygen and get rid of fewer waste products. This is a very uneconomical way of breathing as it uses more muscle power than the deeper and more relaxed abdominal breathing. Pranayama or breath exercises may refer to systems where breath control is worked on in three stages. First is to breathe in from the outside, second is breath retention, and third is to exhale letting go. Working in pranayama allows the practitioner to stretch, expand, or lengthen the breath.

Abdominal breathing is effective breathing. Deep and effective breathing reaches all the way down to the abdomen. The abdomen expands forward, to the sides, and also towards the spine. The breathing movement can be felt all the way down to the pelvic area and up to the top of the lungs. Abdominal breathing has a calming and relaxing effect as we take fewer, but more effective breaths. We absorb more oxygen and release more waste products with each breath. As an added bonus we also add more qi to our system by using abdominal breathing.

Don't use your chest to breathe. Use your abdomen. One teacher used to say that abdominal breathing is like a return to childhood. Abdominal breathing not only makes us breathe like we did when we were children, it can also rejuvenate bodily functions and organs. If you observe the breathing of a baby lying on its back, you can see how he/she breathes in the rhythmic rise and fall of the abdomen as life energy is absorbed. One teacher referred to abdominal breathing as natural breathing and chest breathing as reversed breathing. Using deep breathing regulation is often the first step in controlling the mind movement, then later the mind movement can be controlled by the will of the mind itself.

There are many variations of pranayama that guide the practitioner's awareness, breath, and prana around the body to gain specific results. Examples such as switching the awareness from right to left brain, opening different portions of the lobes of the lungs, internal organ massage, cooling anxiety techniques, warm-up and cleansing techniques, and more.

Fire Path Yogic Qi Gong Breathing

Here is an easy way to learn again how to breathe with your abdomen and receive many health benefits.

1. Sit or stand comfortably.

2. Place your thumbs on your navel. This will put your hands on your lower dan tien.

3. Place the tip of your tongue behind your front teeth. Be sure your tongue is also touching the roof of your mouth.

4. Inhale through your nose. Lead the breath up the Governing Vessel. The breath should take you at least six seconds.

5. Gently hold for two seconds.

6. Lift up and hold the hoi yin.

7. Drop the tongue and exhale through the nose for six seconds. Visualize the warm heart red fire energy descending to the navel.

8. Follow the breath down the Conception Vessel.

Creating The Brass Basin

The brass basin is located in the lower abdomen. The bottom sets on the perineum. The front of the basin is touches the navel and the back of the basin touches the L2-L3 vertebrae. Visualize the basin and place a golden Chi Ball in it. Now, start to spin the ball counter clock-wise. Spinning up the back and down the front.

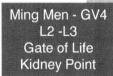

Ming Men - GV4
L2 -L3
Gate of Life
Kidney Point

QiHai - CV6
Sea of Qi
Navel Point, Spleen

Hui Yin - CV1
Meeting of Yin
Gate of Life & Death
Perineum

Sitting Nei Gong—Mixing Kan and Li

The sitting Nei Gong or meditation is a key ingredient in personal cultivation. The main goal of Zen Yoga is cultivating jing, qi, and shen. Jing is the slowest moving energy commonly seen as form. Qi is the energy that animates form, and shen is the consciousness that resides in form. In order to cultivate jing, one must move in a balanced manner using any one of the skillful means such as yoga, tai chi or qi gong. In order for qi to move, one must keep still. Keeping still is also known as meditation or nei gong. Shen or consciousness evolves as qi rises to the upper energy center commonly know as the sixth charka.

Consider this ancient analogy: Visualize a block of ice in the center of the body behind the navel. This block of ice represents jing energy in a frozen and hard state. By moving the body one starts to melt the ice. As the ice melts and heats up, the steam or qi begins to rise. The rising qi ascends up the spine to the head to nourish the shen, inducing illumination and the elevation of one's consciousness.

Be sure to practice sitting meditation after every training session. The following description on meditation is an introductory practice to a life-long study.

Sit comfortably grounding the tailbone, lifting the head and relaxing the shoulders. Let all tension melt away from the body. Place your tongue on the top plate of the mouth. Inhale through the nose leading the breath up the spine. Now keeping the eyes closed look up and visualize the sun with the left eye and the moon with the right eye. Cross the eyes and look to the center of your forehead and mix the sun and moon (kan and li).

The next step is to lead the chi to the lower energy center or second chakra. As you exhale through the nose drop the tongue to touch the bottom plate. Now visualize the golden chi ball you created by mixing the sun and moon descending down the front of the body and resting in the lower energy center. Repeat this process 108 times. Each time you exhale, the golden qi ball should grow, eventually becoming as large as your body.

Now that you have completed your 108 breaths, just sit with no effort and relax for a few moments before standing and completing your meditation. Some people choose to use a mala (108 strung beads) to help them count the breath.

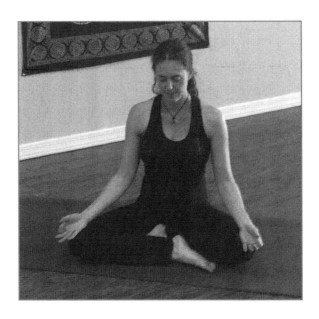

Sitting Nei Gong
Bone Marrow Rejuvenation

Nei gong is simply internal energy work, as wei gong is about our external energy work. The deepest physical energetic work is within the bones. Bones are alive, which is sometimes a surprise. They are filled with spongy marrow in which blood cells are produced. The health of these structures are often seen in strength and vitality, and in Zen Yoga the bones belong to the water element.

A meditation and pranayama exercise for restoring and rejuvenating the bone marrow strength and vitality includes leading, wrapping, and packing prana into the bones.

The concept of bones being a crystalline structure that vibrates indicates the ability to work with its frequency as if tuning a radio to a station. Tune it correctly—get a good result (healthy strong bones); keep it out of tune, get static.

The experience of this practice is taught in Zen Yoga Live (online, phone, and in person).

Sage

The sage training cultivates inner-peace and Zen. Zen means presence.

- ✦ You calm the mind and dissolve the "voice in the head" that is in constant dialog. This calming of the mind and the ability to create "space in between your thoughts" is the key to Zen. Your mind becomes clear, relaxed, yet with razor-like sharpness and focus.

- ✦ The sage knows that "you are not your thoughts" and "you are not your story [or life situation]." Your thoughts are blips of energy that flow through you. There is an "observer" in you that has the ability to watch your thoughts. Unfortunately, this observer mostly lies dormant, and the average person is completely lost in his thoughts and "attached" to her life situation.

- ✦ The sage knows that past and future are just thoughts [blips of energy] and the only moment that is "real" is the now. You stay focused and present in this moment.

- ✦ This of course does not mean that you do not create and design your life. On the contrary, the sage knows cause and effect [karma] and has both the discipline learned during the warrior training and the wisdom learned during the scholar training to engineer and design the lifestyle of his or her choosing.

◆ There is an opposing balance between being fiercely deliberate in your life design and being playful as you "allow this moment to unfold." You, as the sage, are in complete acceptance of the "is-ness" of this moment.

—Blessings

Jason Campbell

Calming the mind to find the sage is from focusing the breath and the mind.

What Is a Mantra?

A mantra is a sound, word, or phrase often repeated in prayer or meditation to express one's basic beliefs. Mantras may pass through direct transmission from teachers to students. Many lineages have song-like repetitions used to connect the mind of the individual to a higher source. Examples would be hymnals, Native American chanting, yogic chanting, rosary prayers and even a repetition of a series of words that keep the mind focused in one direction.

Here are a few popular ones to get you started. Have a look online for pronunciations and meanings. Then pick one that you feel drawn toward. Sit in a quiet place and repeat the mantra (silently or out loud) 108 times.

Om

Gayatri Mantra
Oṁ Bhūr Bhuva~Swah' Tat Savitur varenyam bhargo devasya dhīmahi dhiyo yo naḥ prachodayāt.

Om Mani Padme Hum

Part 11: Pranayama (Qi Gong Breath Work)

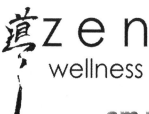

om ma ni pad me hum

Om is a sacred syllable, sometimes translated as "Pure Body"
Mani means "jewel" or "bead"
Padme is the "lotus flower" or "widsom"
Hum refers to the spirit of enlightenment and "unity"

 om = wood

 ma = fire

 ni = earth

 pad = qi

 me = metal

 hum = water

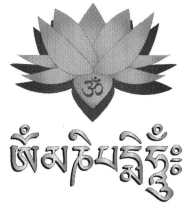

Copyright 2016 Zen Wellness   www.zenwellness.com

Why do Mantra?

Mantra work is valuable on all three levels. On a shen level the consciousness is evoked to connect with the frequency of the words. It's good for the mind to have a pattern of thought to keep it from wandering amongst negative thoughts. This practice protects the mind from its tendency to constantly loop thoughts. A school of thought behind mantra work contains the teaching of vibrations. Each word that is spoken reverberates at least a little in the larynx or voice box. When practicing mantra work, the practitioner expands the vibrations to expand through the entire body thus creating that frequency level to vibrate all of the cells and areas of the body—tuning it if you will—to meet and match the vibration. Cellular structures in the body contain walls and shapes that are imperative to be managed and properly aligned to keep the cell in a good working order. Once cell structure is compromised then the cell no longer is able to provide protection from invaders, let alone do its proper job of taking in nutrients and assimilating the nutrients to repair or build stronger cellular structures. This would be the basis of cancer, which has been said to occur from past resentments. Looping negative thoughts over feelings of being wronged creates stress on a cellular level.

The use of mantra work is now accepted in the psychology field as a portable mind-body-spiritual strategy for managing stress known as mantram repetition in Western culture.

Part 12

Nadis/Meridians The Horary Cycle/ Astrological Twelve

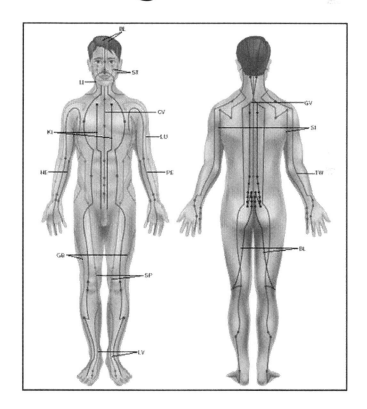

Your Body's Energy Highways

Over five thousand years ago, the ancient Vedas discovered a subtle energy in the body that can't be seen, felt, or found with the five senses. Energy disturbances in the subtle bodies precede the manifestation of abnormal patterns of cellular organization and growth. Matter and energy are two different manifestations of the same primary energetic substance of which everything in the universe is composed, including our physical and subtle bodies. Matter, which vibrates at a very slow frequency, is referred to as *physical* matter. That which vibrates at speeds exceeding light velocity is known as *subtle* matter. Subtle matter is as real as dense or physical matter; its vibratory rate is simply faster. It is believed that two opposite ends of the spectrum—*yin* (the energy of earth), and *yang* (the energy of heaven)—combined with humans to create this vital force.

The Vedas discovered and identified nadis along which this energy travels in the human body. The Chinese took these nadis and arranged them into twelve acupuncture meridians that are like copper traces on an electronic circuit board running throughout the body. They were named by the life function associated with them. To the majority of Western scientists, acupuncture meridians seem like imaginary structures because there are no published anatomical studies of the meridians in orthodox medical journals to substantiate their existence. They prefer to believe that nerve pathways constitute the true mechanism of acupuncture therapy.

Nadis are meridians or highways within the body that energy flows through to deliver and exchange prana around the body. These highways move the prana between the main organs and the prana reservoirs (vessels). There are twelve meridians that are actually connected like a big rubber band stretching through the body and as if painted twelve colors to show twelve segments of the band. The meridians connect and create this circuit. The health of an individual is in direct relation to the elasticity of this "band." The bulk of one's prana resides in one portion of the body—or one organ region at a time. This is a view from TCM, yet Western medicine has also drawn the same conclusion that the body works on one organ at a time. Meridians have been located in the body by Western medicine studies and are said to be filled with synovial fluid, DNA, and stem cells. The prana that travels through the meridians to organs is sometimes impeded or blocked, causing stagnation and imbalance much like a traffic jam on a freeway. When prana does arrive unimpeded to its destination, the prana is able to bring in the new and disperse the old.

Meridians connect specific teeth, organs, tissues, and, in fact, everything in the body. These have been measured and mapped by modern technological methods; *electronically, thermally,* and *radioactively.* Normal skin resistance over a healthy point is 100,000 Ohms. With practice and awareness the meridians can be felt. Through these meridians passes an invisible nutritive energy known to the Chinese as *qi* and the Vedas as *prana*. The energy enters the body through specific acupuncture points and flows to deeper organ structures, bringing life-giving nourishment of a subtle energetic nature. Acupuncture points have unique electrical characteristics which distinguish them from surrounding skin. These acupuncture points exist along the meridians. These points are electromagnetic in character and consist of small palpable spots that can be located by hand, with micro-electrical voltage meters and with muscle testing when they are functioning abnormally.

These five hundred points, mapped and used for centuries to optimize human performance, are connections between the positive and negative meridians and functions of the body including internal organs and muscles. These points are useful not only in treatment but also in diagnosis of disease states. Subtle magnetic qi currents flowing through the acupuncture meridians are not electrical in nature, but they are able to induce secondary electrical fields that create measurable changes at the physical cellular level through the induction of secondary electrical fields.

These induced electrical fields are translated into DC-current interactions from the higher energy meridians into the physical body and affect primary bio-electronic processes that provide and maintain coherence within the physical-cellular structure. When the flow of life energy to a particular organ is deficient or unbalanced, patterns of cellular disruption occur. Imbalances in the meridians can be detected by feeling the pulses, but this ability can take up to twenty years to develop proficiently.

The Meridian Cycle

Meridians are classified yin or yang on the basis of the direction in which they flow on the surface of the body. Meridians interconnect deep within the torso but we will work with the part that is on the surface and is accessible to touch techniques. Yang energy flows from the sun, and yang meridians run from the fingers to the face or from the face to the feet. Yin energy, from the earth, flows from the feet to the torso, and from the torso along the inside (yin side) of the arms to the fingertips. Since the meridian flow is actually one continuous unbroken flow, the energy flows in one definite direction, and from one meridian to another in a well determined order. Since there is no beginning or end to this flow, the order can be represented as a wheel. The flow around the wheel follows the meridian lines on the body in this order:

1. From torso to fingertip (along inside of arm—yin).
2. From fingertip to face (along outside/back of arm—yang).
3. From face to feet (along outside of leg—yang).
4. From feet to torso (along inside of the leg—yin).

Three times through this four-step process covers the Twelve Major Meridians.

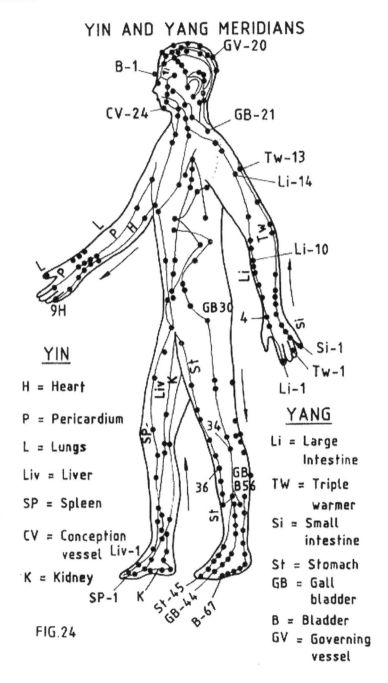

FIG. 24

Earth
Spleen
Stomach

Spleen Meridian
(Earth Element)

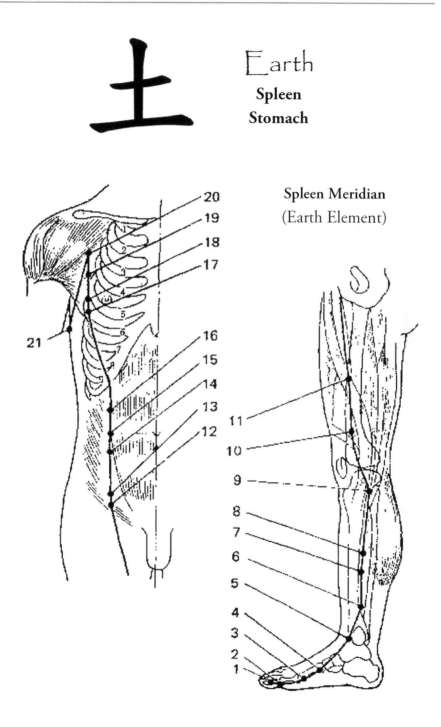

Zen Yoga: Theory, Postures, and Remedies

Fire
Heart
Small Intestine

Heart Meridian
(Fire Element)

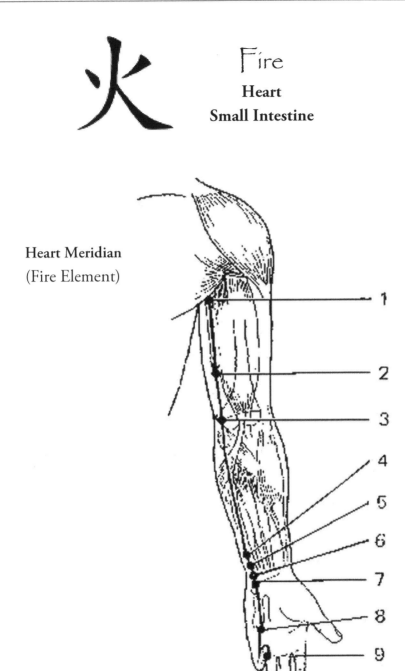

Fire
Heart
Small Intestine

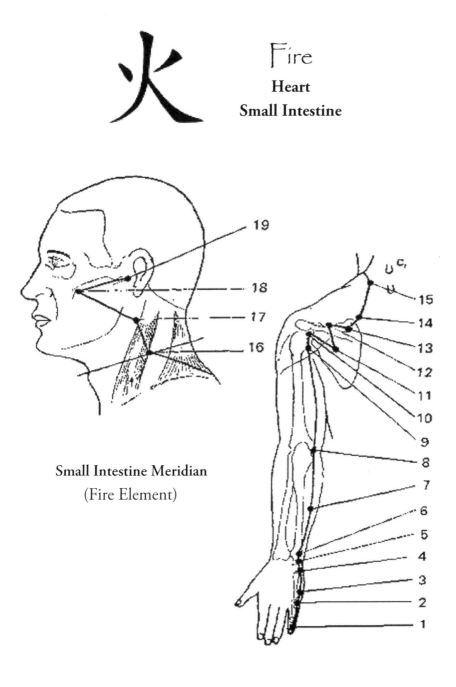

Small Intestine Meridian
(Fire Element)

Water
**Kidneys
Bladder**

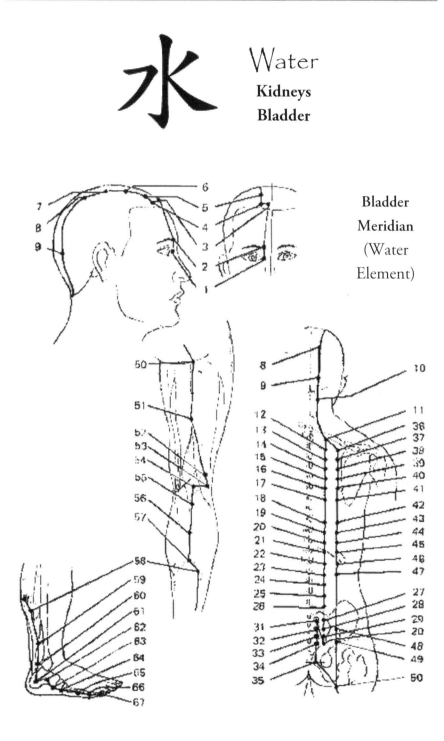

**Bladder
Meridian
(Water
Element)**

Part 12: Nadis/Meridians, The Horary Cycle/Astrological Twelve

Water
Kidneys
Bladder

Kidney Meridian
(Water Element)

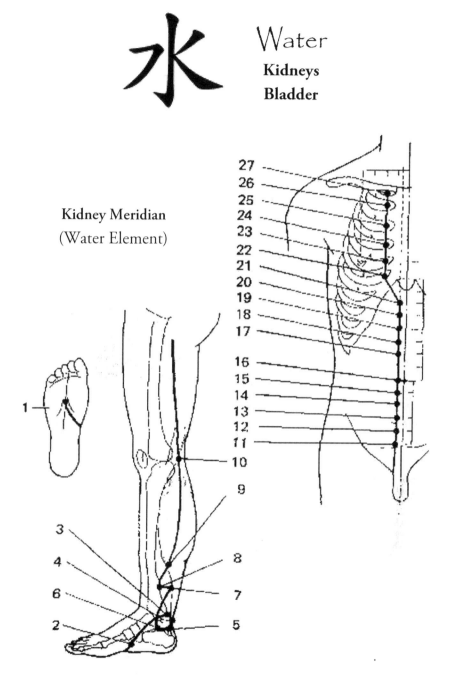

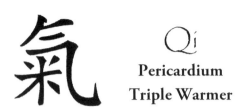

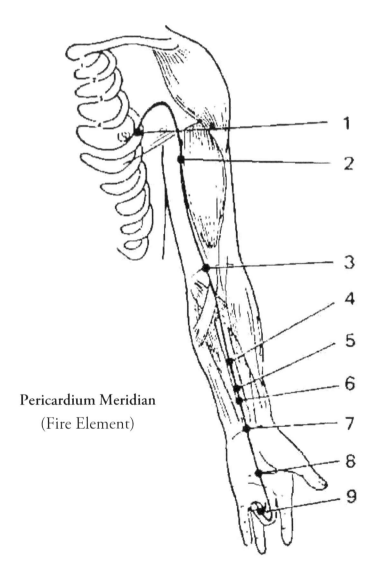

Pericardium Meridian
(Fire Element)

Part 12: Nadis/Meridians, The Horary Cycle/Astrological Twelve

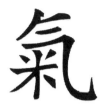

Qí
Pericardium
Triple Warmer

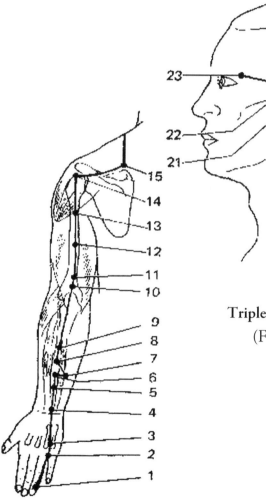

Triple Heater Meridian
(Fire Element)

Wood
Gallbladder
Liver

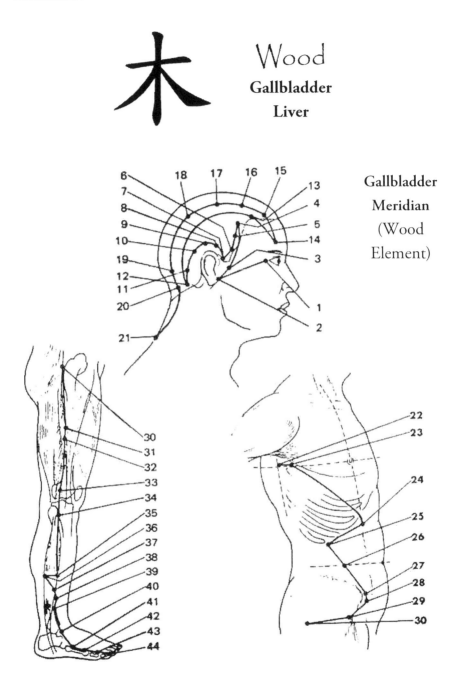

Gallbladder Meridian (Wood Element)

Part 12: Nadis/Meridians, The Horary Cycle/Astrological Twelve

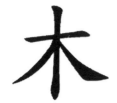

Wood
Gallbladder
Liver

Liver Meridian
(Wood Element)

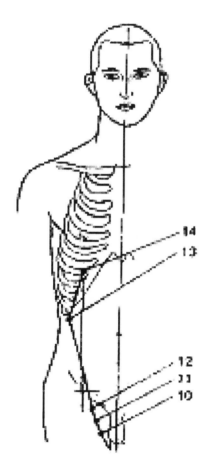
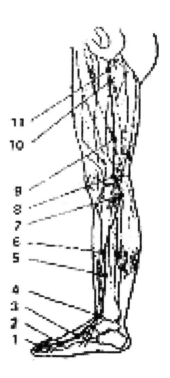

What Is the Horary Cycle?

The horary cycle is the cycle in which energy flows around the body and through each organ. As Western medicine has found that each organ holds dominant blood at specific times of day, the Eastern understanding has known for many years that the bulk of the energy or blood resides in one organ at a time. During the peak time for that organ, the body does its repair work for that organ on all three levels while processing the corresponding emotions related to that organ's elemental nature. Below is the clock in which a specific organ and body part is at high tide. First is to simply be aware of the timing, then to learn how to assist the processes. The time is in relation to your current time zone.

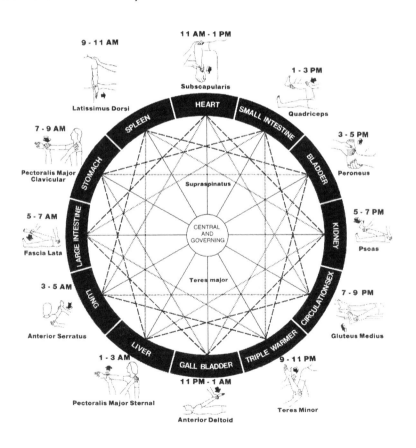

Part 12: Nadis/Meridians, The Horary Cycle/Astrological Twelve

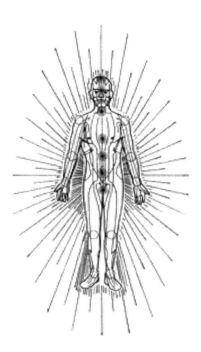

Meridians are present at birth. However, they develop in sets of four during the first months of life. The first set develops in months one to four. The second set develops in months four through eight. The final set develops in months eight to twelve.

First one becomes aware of their existence, then how to aid their flow. When impeded, they are disturbed as well as the organ to which they flow. Optimal flow appears as balanced unimpeded flow that is neither excessive nor deficient.

Meridians run along the muscle bellies and therefore may be addressed by physical movement and manipulation. Each posture will address specific meridians.

Each meridian belongs to one of the elements, and has each of the Five Elements within them. The liver meridian, for example, belongs to the wood element, yet along the meridian there are points that belong to wood, fire, earth, metal, and water. So there would be a wood of wood point, a fire of wood, and earth of wood, and so on. If there is too much fire in the wood liver meridian, one might activate the water of wood point to calm the excessive fire.

The chart below details the points along the meridians.

YIN YANG	WEAK YANG	STRONG YANG	CENTER 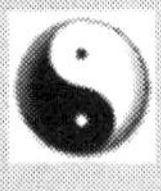	WEAN YIN	STRONG YIN
ELEMENT	WOOD	FIRE	EARTH	METAL	WATER

Five Element Points of the 12 Meridians

YIN	WELL	SPRING	STREAM	RIVER	SEA
ELEMENT	WOOD	FIRE	EARTH	METAL	WATER
LU	11	10	9	8	5
SP	1	2	3	5	9
HT	9	8	7	4	3
KI	1	2	3	7	10
PC	9	8	7	5	3
LR	1	2	3	4	8

YANG	WELL	SPRING	STREAM	RIVER	SEA
ELEMENT	METAL	WATER	WOOD	FIRE	EARTH
LI	1	2	3	5	11
ST	45	44	43	41	36
SI	1	2	3	5	8
BL	67	66	65	60	40
TW	1	2	3	6	10
GB	44	43	41	38	34

Astrology—Twelve Animals

Astrology = Astral + Study (Study of the Stars)
Zodiac = Zoo + Circle (Circle of Animals)

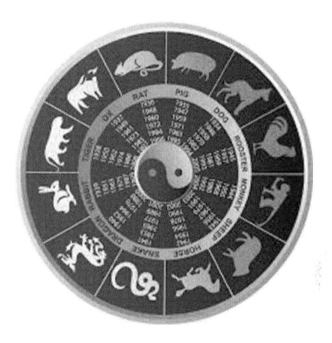

In videos and snapshots of the sky's vast universe, within the frame of the picture the planets and solar systems move about the universe with the backdrop of stars. As all planets move at their own pace and orbits, some may be close, far, scattered, aligned, and so on. The vastness of our sky's window to the universe gives a 360-degree view as our planet revolves. This 360-degree view is like a round pizza divided into twelve slices. Even with the same ingredients all around the pizza, each piece will vary. The sky view of the universe seen with a 360-degree view is also divided in to twelve slices (or houses). Each of these twelve are given a description of what is found within that house. Since the planets move around our 360-degree view, they naturally travel into different houses and reside there for a period of time. Planets move to and fro and sometimes seem to spin backwards when apexing. These movements of planets in our sky's universal pool create ripples that affect all other planets in the universal pool. Effects can be positive or negative, weak or strong, kind or harsh to the observer. Yet within the universal view they are just effects. Not good or bad, they're simply movements along the way of the ongoing creation of our universe.

From a human's standpoint, the understanding of a planet's movement is paramount—such as with farming and understanding which planets bring birth and growth, and which are barren. Knowing planting times assists in the harvest quality and quantity. This understanding apply's to every aspect of life since life is simply the unfolding of a Five Elemental process always starting from wood through water. This Five Elemental life within our planet is placed in the universal pool with the other eight planets in our solar system.

Astrology can help, but it is not the whole answer. When looking objectively at one's individual nature, we see vast influences on ourselves and our lives. We are a mixing pot of a variety of components that includes astrology, DNA (heredity and ancestors), geographical location and environment, social class, economic level, religion and belief structure, physical appearance and ability, health, race, and gender (to name a few).

Astrology is not classified as magic and an astrologer should not claim to have magical powers. Its best use is simply for viewing a person or entity's timeline to see how it is affecting the person or situation.

Astrology is a tool to uncover bits of one's total character similar to psychology, analysis, hypnotherapy, healing, numerology, tarot, *I Ching* or any other number of means for developing self-knowledge, yet still without the complete picture.

One of the best use for astrology is as a tool for co-existence. When we can get a glimpse of our nature and of those around us, we can view where conflicts or differences of personalities might clash or align. By knowing whom we are dealing with around us, it may help to dissolve the personal nature in which we find differences. At the end of the day our differences do not make one person correct and the other wrong (well not always), instead they may offer a glimpse of where the other is standing in relation to the object being viewed.

The arrangement of the planets, the stars in their current backdrop, the gravitational ebb and tide of the moon, and our sun all create different scenes as they orbit. Watching each planet's own orbital time (how long it takes to go around the sun once), where it goes on its journey, what was affecting it along the way, what interactions between other planets, moons, stars, and nodes—the results of these interactions are recorded and studied. Repetitive patterns within history allow us to take a snapshot of the sky at any time and see where it is in the transiting pattern. This is the foundation of astrology.

Co-existence using the astrology tool is sought by many searching for answers in life. Answers can be found, but be cautious in having no ill intentions when seeking an answer. Laws of karma encourage the cultivation of higher aspirations, not harmful ones.

All forms are matter vibrating and emitting a frequency. Planets, stars, the sun and moon emit a frequency. When two items are close, they can affect the other's field of frequency. More recently the relationships of planets, moons, sun, and stars has been seen as a web with cords connecting everything, which astronomers witnessed when viewing a distant quasar that illuminated a filament of the cosmic web. On earth we feel the effects of other frequencies in the universe that have changed.

Often astrology is used for seeing the sky map at the time of a particular event, such as for the birth chart of a person, business, governmental institution, relationship, and so on. There are multiple methods for interpreting a birth chart. Ultimately the root self will be expressed with accurate interpretation.

Birth charts in Chinese astrology may be drawn through the Four Pillars: the sun (year) pillar, moon (month) pillar, day pillar, and hour pillar. A pillar is an image (or hexagram) of two trigrams stacked, divided into pre-heaven and post-heaven designations. The information gives a look into what the life is predisposed to from our family and our soul's past, and our outlook for how the life will unfold while in form—the fate of the life's expression. Of course this is augmented by free will to give way for destiny to be attained.

The sun pillar describes how the life expression is seen by the outside world—your personality, your most noticeable and important characteristics, your methods for making decisions, positive and negative personality traits, qualities you like and dislike. The sign shown here is then viewed with the effect of its associated element. The moon, day, and hour pillars show emotional, familial, and financial propensities.

Example Four Pillar designation with corresponding animal signs:

Year—Earth Pig, Month—Wood Rat,
Day—Water Goat, Hour—Fire Monkey.

What are the Twelve Chinese Astrological Signs? (Twelve Earthly Branches)

The traditional Spring Festival story says that Buddha invited the animals to celebrate the New Year with him, and when they arrived, he named a year for each of them, then gave the people born in each animal's year a part of that animal's power and personality. The order of the animal's arrival occurred as follows:

Rat

Ox

Tiger

Cat/Rabbit

Dragon

Snake

Horse

Goat/Sheep

Monkey

Rooster

Dog

Pig

Five Elements for Years—What Element Are You?

The year of birth in which you were born corresponds to one of the Five Elements. An easy way for determining your element is to consider the last numeral in your year of birth and find your element below:

> 0 or 1: Metal
> 2 or 3: Water
> 4 or 5: Wood
> 6 or 7: Fire
> 8 or 9: Earth

If you were born in 1977, for example, your element is Fire; if you were born in 1950, your element is Metal, and so forth

As to the elemental influence, "wood-related" industries like fashion, education, advisory services, furniture, timber, and plantations, for example, would thrive in a wood year.

The 60-Year Cycle

The Five Elements form the Ten Heavenly Stems of Chinese Astrology when viewed with their yin and yang aspects:

1. Yang Wood	2. Yin Wood
3. Yang Fire	4. Yin Fire
5. Yang Earth	6. Yin Earth
7. Yang Metal	8. Yin Metal
9. Yang Water	10. Yin Water

The rotation through the Twelve Animal signs and their corresponding Five Elements completes a sixty-year cycle. Five (for each of the elements) x twelve (for each of the animal signs) = sixty years.

The Twelve Animal's Influence on Personality

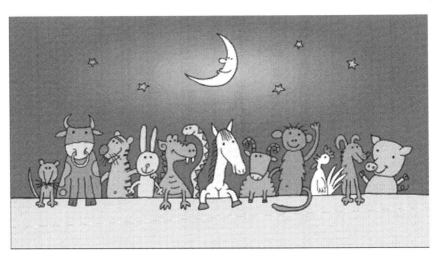

The Rat contains the element water. Basic characteristics include adaptability, intelligence, charm, social ability, artistic qualities, and quick wit. The rat partners well with both the monkey and dragon.

The Ox contains the element earth and is known for its characteristics of loyalty, thoroughness, reliability, strength, steadiness, reasonableness, and determination. The ox partners well with roosters and snakes.

The Tiger contains the element wood and has attributes that include courage, enthusiasm, competence, leadership, ambition, and charisma. The tiger partners well with dog and horse.

The Rabbit contains the element wood and has aspects that include empathy, trustworthiness, modesty, sincerity, diplomacy, and social ability. Rabbits are known for being caretakers and partner well with both the pig and goat.

The Dragon contains the element earth and is know for its flexibility, luck, eccentricity, artistry, charisma, and spiritualism. The dragon partners well with monkey and rat.

The Snake contains the element fire and is known for its intelligence, organizational skills, intuitiveness, attentiveness, elegance, decisiveness, and philosophical nature. Snakes partner well with oxen and roosters.

The Horse contains the element fire and has individual traits that include loyalty, adaptability, ambition, courage, adventure, strength, and intelligence. It partners well with both the tiger and dog.

The Goat contains the element earth and has characteristics that include craftiness, tastefulness, warmth, elegance, intuition, charm, calmness, and sensitivity. Goats partner well with rabbits and pigs.

The Monkey contains the element metal and is known for having charm, a quick wit, luck, adaptability, versatility, intellect, liveliness, and a bright and airy personality. The monkey partners well with both the rat and the dragon.

The Rooster contains the element metal and has characteristics that include energy, honesty, intelligence, flexibility, confidence, diversity and a flamboyant personality. The rooster partners well with the ox and the snake.

The Dog contains the element earth and is known for its characteristics that include social grace, courage, loyalty, diligence, adaptability, steadiness, intellect, and a lively personality. The dog partners well with the horse and tiger.

The Pig contains the element water and is known for its honor, determination, philanthropy, sincerity, optimism, and sociable personality. Pigs partner well with rabbits and sheep.

To view possible life expressions for any given astrological sign, examine the animal's propensities with an undertone of the elemental influence. Charting the astrology for the individual life expression is also applied to the *I Ching (Book of Changes)* as each animal and element goes to a specific image of the 64 Hexagrams in the *I Ching*. There are many texts to reference that show the animal and elemental indications. Years progress through each animal in the order of creation with the elements moving through their yin and yang designations. Meaning, a yang-wood Rat year would be followed by a yin-wood Ox year.

You can calculate what animal and element a year will be if you know some root year, such as 1960 being a Metal Rat year. Twelve years from then, 1972, will be another Rat year, and the element will be the next in sequence from metal, making 1972 a Water Rat year. The Wood Rat year will then be 1984, Fire Rat is 1996, and 2008 the Earth Rat year. Metal Rat returns after sixty years, which will be 2020.

The elemental rotation stays in each element for two years, first being yang then yin. With Metal Rat of 1960 being yang, the next year 1961 is yin Metal and Ox. Then 1962 would be yang water, and 1963 yin water, and so on.

As much as the astrology may give an insider's view to the life's expression, it may also show the flavor of each year by revealing what the energies are in that year's animal and elemental expression. Starting with the months (which change with the moon, not the gregorian calendar), the Rat moon covers the time of the winter solstice, and moves forward from there to an Ox moon. Chinese New year follows the Moon, while the Chinese Zodiac follows the Sun. Therefore, the Chinese New Year does not start on the beginning of the Zodiac cycle, but instead on the budding of the Spring moon coinciding with the moving into the Tiger moon (the most spring-like creature, of course).

The days revolve in a microcycle of the sixty years as a sixty-day rotation—meaning, Wood Rat day to Wood Ox day, and so on.

The hours move through the animals with each hour covering a two-hour period (one hour being yang, and the other yin), just like the way meridian energy flow resides in each organ for two hours a day. The element of the animal progressively moves forward through the creative cycle as well. If it is the Wood Goat one day, the next day at that time period will be Fire Goat, then the following day that time period will have Earth Goat characteristics and so forth.

The hours between 11:00 p.m. and 1:00 a.m. belong to the Rat and the gall bladder; 1:00 a.m. to 3:00 a.m. belong to the Ox and liver; 3:00 a.m. to 5:00 a.m. belong to Tiger, po and lungs; 5:00 a.m. to 7 a.m. belong to Rabbit and large intestine; and so on.

Time	Animal	Organ
11pm-1am	Rat	Gall Bladder
1am-3am	Ox	Liver
3am-5am	Tiger	Lungs
5am-7am	Cat	Large Intestine
7am-9am	Dragon	Stomach
9am-11am	Snake	Spleen
11am-1pm	Horse	Heart
1pm-3pm	Goat	Small Intestine
3pm-5pm	Monkey	Bladder
5pm-7pm	Rooster	Kidney
7pm-9pm	Dog	Pericardium
9pm-11pm	Pig	Triple Warmer

Note: Although there are many lineages of interpretation for how to read astrology patterns, they all tend to say the same thing, just with different words. Vedic and Western astrologies do not use the animal signs mentioned above, instead they use the zodiac that we are probably more familiar with such as Aquarius, Capricorn, Gemini, Cancer,

Sagittarius, etc. These are constellations that live and hold a particular part of the sky. The sun travels through these parts of the sky throughout the year shining directly on one of these constellations at a time. Often referred to as one's "Sun Sign" in a birth chart. The moon and other planets move around the constellations as well, so when a snapshot in time is taken of the planets' positions in relation to the constellations this would form a horoscope. Also, each animal/element combination belongs to one of the sixty *I Ching* images.

The 64 Parts of a Life's Story

Although one's personal astrology gives a snapshot of their life, we all go through the same series of events or phases. These phases are the front-to-back story of the *I Ching* itself and apply to any life path, whether for a person, business, or so on. Trigrams are stacked on top of each other and called images. This is the foundation of the *I Ching,* or *Book of Changes,* that give examples of how time, energy, and matter move throughout life's expressions. When the Eight Trigrams are stacked in all different possible arrangements there are then a total of sixty-four possibilities. Each of the sixty-four images have been given a name. The heaven trigram over heaven (heaven doubled), for example, may be called "The Creative," while earth over earth may be named "The Receptive."

Each of the sixty-four images is yet another pointer to the type of energy and movement that is occurring. Remember not to get caught up in a single word for the image, as translators of the *I Ching* will offer a variety of words to assist the observer in seeing a balanced view of the image's wisdom teaching. Each of the sixty-four images are constructed around a wheel (360 degrees), each taking up about six degrees and having a direction assigned to them determined by the amount of yin or yang within the image. The Yang Family images begin at the returning of the light just at the winter solstice and build in yang energy until the apex of the summer solstice shown with all yang lines. Then the yin family is predominant, beginning at the summer solstice until the apex of the Yin Family at the winter solstice shown with all yin lines.

The influence how much yin and yang energy in the space is comparable to inhalation and exhalation. Are you expanding or contracting, receiving or letting go? Heavy yin in the space lends itself to contraction and inward movement, as opposed to heavy yang lending itself to expansion and outward movement. This, of course, is a moving target and is mixed like a chess board in play (64 squares with equal yin and yang).

I Ching for Divination and Contemplation

Contemplating the *I Ching* could easily consume most of one's lifetime. The subject is vast and deep for personal and social morality. By reading and contemplating the *I Ching* daily, year after year, the seeker slowly uncovers the natural changes of environment and life. On a simple side, the yin and yang patterns show the amount of light (yang/sunlight) throughout the year, as well as the darkness (yin), aiding the seeker to harmonize with the light and dark seasons by matching lifestyle variances with nature and the heavens.

Below is an example of the *I Ching* wheel. There are many ways to use the *I Ching* for divination, but be cautious and sincere when consulting the oracle and interpreting its guidance.

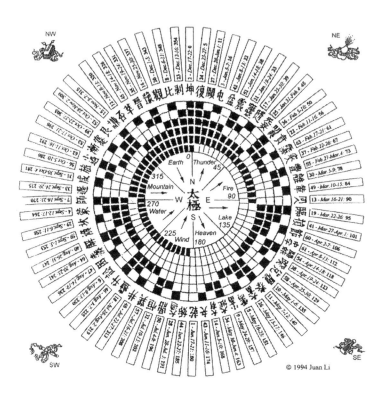

© 1994 Juan Li

Open-ended questions of eight words or less work best. When the question is formed and meditated upon, you may use three coins or the fifty yarrow sticks as a medium to bring forth the answer from the subconscious mind.

A simple way of using coins is to count heads as 3, and tails as 2. Toss the three coins together, take the sum, and repeat five more times for a total of six lines. Start from the bottom line and up, and inside the wheel and out.

COIN COMBOS	NUMBER	LINE
3 Heads	9	——○——
2 Heads, 1 Tail	8	—— ——
1 Head, 2 Tails	7	————
3 Tails	6	——✕——

There is significance to lines that change. There are two yin and two yang changing lines. One of the yin is steady, the other is changing. Same with the yang. If there is a changing line in your answer, the corresponding line it changes into is significant.

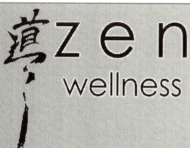

Zen Yoga Program Guide

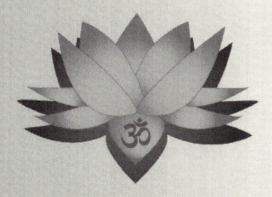

For information and application
call 623-537-9443
info@zenwellness.com
www.zenwellness.com

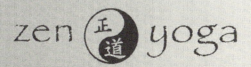

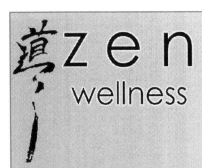

Zen Yoga 200-hour Local or Long Distance Training with Optional Certification Program

*Scholarships Available

This program is designed to meet & exceed the requirements for certification by the Yoga Alliance as a Level 1 Zen Yoga Instructor.

Two hundred hours of documented formal training.

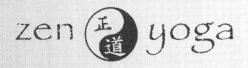

Curriculum

1. Prana & the Golden Qi Ball
   1. Yin-Yang theory
   2. Creating the brass basin
   3. Finding the three hearts
   4. Opening the small circuit
   5. Learning Pranayama

2. Zen Wellness Five Element Zen Yoga
   1. Five element theory
   2. Using the Zen Wellness elemental healing sounds
   3. Zen Wellness five elemental yoga
   4. Zen Wellness five elemental protocols
   5. The three treasures of the Tao: Jing-chi-shen or Vata-Pitta-Kapha

3. Zen Wellness Nine Gates Zen Yoga
   1. What are the nine gates?
   2. Introduction to the twelve meridians
   3. Three hearts and nine gates Zen Yoga. (muscle tendon changing)
   4. Three hearts and nine gates acute Zen Yoga (sitting practice)
   5. Man, heaven and earth meridian breathing
   6. Principles of alignment
   7. Anatomy and physiology

4. Zen Wellness 8-Vessels Zen Yoga Qigong
   1. Introduction to the eight vessels
   2. Opening the eight vessels Zen Yoga Qigong
   3. Filling the eight vessels Zen Yoga Qigong
   4. Introduction to the eight trigrams
   5. The seven dimensions of consciousness or chakras
   6. 8 limbs of Yoga

5. Zen Wellness Bone Marrow Nei Gong
   1. What is bone marrow nei gong?
   2. Iron shirt chi gong
   3. Introduction to Ching Chi nei gong
   4. Bone marrow breathing nei gong
   5. Bone tapping nei gong

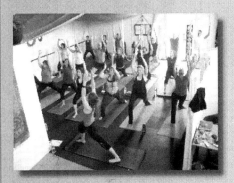

For information and application call 623-537-9443

Copyright 2016 Zen Wellness   www.zenwellness.com

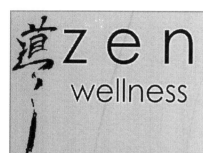

Zen Yoga 200-hour Local or Long Distance Training with Optional Certification Program

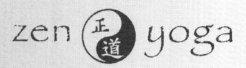

Home Study Qualification

200-hours total documented training:
- 75 hours Learning the Mechanics of Mind and Body Home study - you will learn this through our books and vlogs
- 75 hours documented home study and physical practice of the 5-Element Zen Yoga & Qigong Curriculum
- 25 hours of science of teaching (with Certified Zen Wellness Facility)
- 25 hours practicum and clinic work teaching (with Certified Zen Wellness Facility)
- Upon completion and passing the Instructor exam you will be recognized as a **Zen Yoga 200 Hour Instructor**

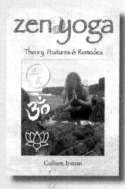

Zen Yoga is a part of the Master's Apprentice program within Zen Wellness.

Zen Yoga 200 hour training includes:

- Zen Yoga: Theory, Postures & Remedies Book
- Secrets for Living Forever Young Book
- Extensive online support via videos, texts, audio teachings, chat and more.

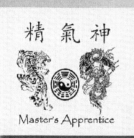

See website for details
www.zenwellness.com

The Zen Yoga® program is the result of studying yoga, martial, medical and spiritual Chi Gong with many grandmasters and masters from around the world. The goal of all of the yoga disciplines is to create a balance of life force energy or chi to enhance the long-term quality of life.

For information and application call 623-537-9443

Copyright 2016 Zen Wellness   www.zenwellness.com

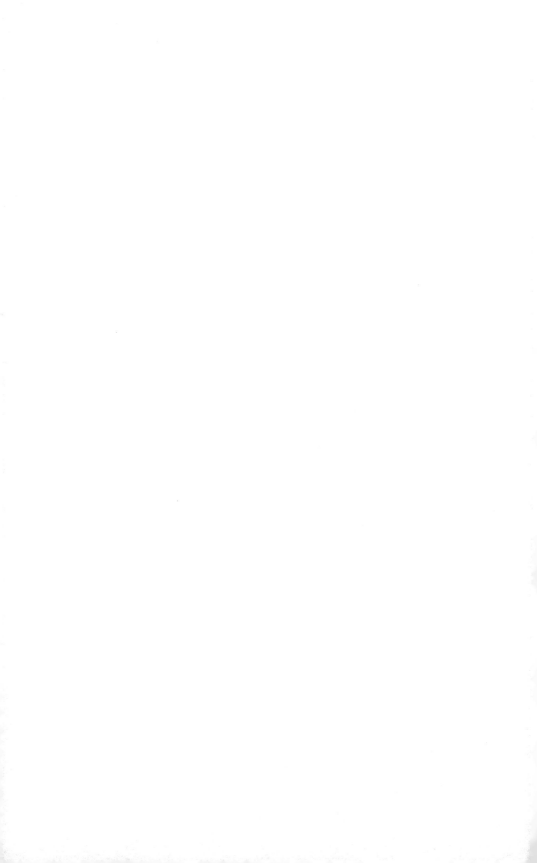

Made in the USA
Middletown, DE
18 July 2018